ADVANCE PRAISE FOR

Deadline Fitness

"Deadline Fitness is simply one of the best and smartest workout books on the market. It's obvious why Hollywood stars turn to Gina when they need to get in shape fast!"

—Jonny Bowden, PhD, CNS board certified nutritionist and bestselling author of *The 150 Healthiest Foods on Earth*

"Gina is an internationally recognized author who uniquely blends art with science. *Deadline Fitness* offers practical ways for the reader to successfully reach his or her individual fitness goals. I enjoy how the book leads the reader through different phases and timelines for a variety of personal fitness objectives and then brings it home to permanent lifestyle changes. Gina applies exercise science for the individual in an effective way, better than anyone I know!"

—Jay Shiner, CSCS, Strength & Conditioning Coach for the Baltimore Orioles

"Gina Lombardi's extensive and thought-out approach to making weight loss healthy is a slam dunk."

—David Evangelista, TV personality and beauty/fashion contributor

"If you have an upcoming event that requires you to improve your fitness and health and look your best, then this is the book for you. It is written simply, and you will have no trouble understanding the concepts and successfully reaching your goals. This book addresses all aspects of health, including workouts, diet plans, and ways to manage stress. Gina's comprehensive plan will allow you to meet your fitness deadline in the most healthy and enjoyable way possible."

—Jaynie Bjornaraa, PhD, MPH, PT, SCS, ATC, CSCS

"Fitness dynamo Gina Lombardi hits a home run with her sensational new book *Deadline Fitness,* featuring individualized programs that will help you lose weight and feel better fast!"

—Jose Antonio, PhD, CEO of the International Society of Sports Nutrition

"Gina Lombardi's *Deadline Fitness* is dead on. With obesity reaching epidemic proportions and families struggling with finding the time to maintain a healthy lifestyle, *Deadline Fitness* provides real-life stories with real-life solutions. Gina's plan breaks down chapters into timelines with realistic goals, solution-driven information, and a healthy dose of motivation. Whether you want to look or feel better, *Deadline Fitness* will set you up for long-term success."

—Carole Tomko, Executive Vice President Discovery Channel USA

Deadline Fitness

Deadline Fitness

Tone Up and Slim Down When Every Minute Counts

GINA LOMBARDI

with Linda Villarosa

WILEY

John Wiley & Sons, Inc.

To my parents, Dr. Joseph and Veglia Lombardi,
who, with the hand of God,
made all things possible for me

Contents

Acknowledgments

It was quite an undertaking to condense my sixty thousand hours of experience in the fitness field into sixty thousand words, but here is the result of my effort. May no one go unnoticed who helped me, listened to me, taught me, changed my mind, told me I couldn't, told me I could, told me I should, challenged me, or encouraged me. You have all made me a better person. Here's to every one of you.

An extraspecial thanks to my fabulous husband, Kevin, for his endless encouragement and for carrying the load while I was glued to my desk chair, and to my spectacular son, Gunnar Cruise Sizemore, whose gentle sweetness made the sacrifices worthwhile. Thank you, Gunnar, for rolling your Hot Wheels cars under my office door. For the record, I already knew you were there.

To my incredibly patient agent and friend, Manie Baron, for all the hand-holding, good jokes, and great advice. You da man!

To the awesome John Wiley & Sons publishing company, especially Tom Miller and Dan Crissman.

To Linda Villarosa, for your editing skills, patience, and finesse.

To my clients: to *everyone*, past, present, and future, whom I have worked with, thank you for the opportunity to serve you, to laugh and cry with you, to help you, and to learn from you. You are the reason I am in this profession.

A special thanks to Vatche, Mayda, and Joanna Meguerdichian; Bonnie, Barry, and Crispin; Susan; Jack; the lovely Catherine Bell; the sassy Sally "Mustang Sally" Pressman; Kathryn Gordon; Deirdre Waitt and John Mendoza; Romina; Talar; Kristie; John, Esther, and Christine; and Chris Beetem for your great stories.

To my colleagues: the National Strength and Conditioning Association (NSCA) and the entire staff in Colorado Springs, whose dedication to human performance is second to none; the International Society of Sports Nutrition, specifically Dr. Jose Antonio and Dr. Douglas Kalman for answering endless questions at all hours of the day and night for me; Dr. Thomas Baechle and Roger Earle for inviting me to serve the NSCA in developing what has become the finest, most widely recognized certification for personal trainers; Peter and Kathie Davis; Dr. Jonny Bowden and his dogs, all of whom are brilliant; Dr. Uzzi Reiss—my genius friend, I will always adore your brilliance and courage to do what everyone else is afraid of doing; Jacqueline Stenson, MSNBC, Beth Dreher and *Health* magazine for all the great opportunities to disseminate solid information on the Web and in print; Dr. William Kramer; the NSCA Japan: Ryoji, Sam and Reiko, Mayumi, Naoko, Naho and Nobuko; "Special K," Shelly, and Chris Mansolillo at Exercise TV; Fuze Beverage; the University of Pennsylvania and the University of California, Los Angeles, for an outstanding education.

A very special thanks to Carole Tomko at the Discovery Channel for allowing me to disseminate on the airwaves.

To my family and friends: the Lombardis: Marc, Velia (MFS), Joe, Dave, Eric, and Chris, along with Elise, Tony, Cathy, Gina, Veronica, and Wendy. And Xander, Livi, Gia, Nicolas, Devan, Matthew, Erica, Louie, Brittney, and Justin. Isn't it our childhood that makes us who we are? To Woodlea Road and beyond!

The Sizemores—Jeff, Luisa, Jordan, Logan, Davit, and Wanda, John, Sandy, Lucille, and Henry Brown, and everyone in the holler.

To my buddies: my oldest, yet ageless, friend, Adrienne "A-Baby" Gallo, thank God for gymnastics class at Radnor High; Rick and Richie; Susan Wood Duncan, what would I do without your amazing friendship and constant great advice! Cathy Assetto and Caryn Fallon; through thick and thin, Rosie DeSanctis and the *whole* family; Ifer; Gina "Gigi" Turner, for your friendship and great abs and Corey Turner for allowing the world to see Gina's great abs in this book; Deb Gurin; Firefly; Bridget, Jared, and Dylan Wheelock; Sarah and Veronica Graveline; Julie and Romeo, Marji and Geoff—for all your advice and unconditional friendship; Gil, Ruth, and Sophie. BETO: the talented Jared Bentley.

To Dabling Harward, my "monochromatic friend," who worked countless hours to shoot and edit the beautiful photos for this book; and to the artistic Jane Koo.

To my patient teachers: especially Shihan Mark Parra, who spends hours allowing me to kick and punch him; Benny "the Jet" Urquidez; Shihan Dennis Swarthout; and Master Tak Kubota.

To Roger Schwab, the founder of Main Line Health and Fitness in Bryn Mawr, Pennsylvania, who taught me first and taught me right.

Introduction

When I moved to Los Angeles from the East Coast, I was thrilled to have the opportunity to work in the entertainment industry. As I was studying and building my fitness business, my day job was as an assistant account executive at a Beverly Hills public relations firm. I spent lots of time with up-and-comers as well as with the most established actors, and after a while, I started to notice that every time any of them had a major audition or had just landed a role, they'd fly into a crazy panic about how their bodies looked. Time was short, and they needed to lose weight, lean out, and shape up fast. But none of them had any idea how to do it. Back then personal trainers were hard to come by—unlike today.

I clearly remember a beautiful British actress who had just landed a starring role on *Star Trek: The Next Generation*. She was probably 15 or 20 pounds overweight, but had no idea how to handle it. So she went on the latest herbal diet pill and basically starved herself into thinness. I thought, *There's got to be a better way to help these well-meaning people get what they need without putting them in danger.*

I realized that if I could come up with a whole plan—diet *and* exercise—for these actors and actresses, I'd hit a home run. So taking advantage of my science background, I created a formula. Using the assessment tools, nutritional knowledge, and training experience I had gained at the University of Pennsylvania, at UCLA, and in the real world, I devised data-driven, science-based eating and exercise programs, tailor-made to the individual client. Given that I was working with celebrities, who are notoriously fickle, I knew that my plan had to be foolproof. If it didn't work 100 percent of the time, I'd be out of a job.

Three years ago, after more than two decades in the business, it finally hit me that I had succeeded. I was sitting at home on a Friday night, nine months pregnant and feeling as big as a house; my labor was scheduled to be induced the following day. At around noon, the phone rang. It was a New York soap opera actor in a total panic. He was in LA after landing a lead role as a Navy lieutenant on *JAG*, a hit CBS military drama. In his first episode, two weeks away, he had to do a scene on the beach with his shirt off. He felt he was a little "soft," and his costar had told him to call me. "Everybody goes to her. She's the one you want if you need to get ready fast," his costar had said.

"I'm going into the hospital tomorrow—in twenty-four hours—to deliver my son," I said, looking down at my oversize belly. But the guy wouldn't take no for an answer. "I'll come to *your* house . . . tonight," he insisted.

A few hours later, he was at my door, eager to do whatever I might tell him. Although he was great-looking and certainly *not* over-weight, he needed a leaner look, more definition. To the rest of us mortals, it might have seemed like overkill, but I understood his thinking. After all, millions of people, as well as the network executives, would be looking at him. I spent the next hour taking his measurements, doing questionnaires, checking his blood pressure, measuring his body fat—all my normal procedures. I had to have him stand on a chair because I couldn't bend down to measure his thighs and calves. I stayed up until midnight detailing his program of specific eating recommendations, weight training, and cardio. A few hours later, I clicked Send on the e-mail and it landed in his in-box.

Aah . . . another deadline met; another life saved. Ten days later he had reached his goal: he had lost body fat, improved definition, and shot the last eight episodes of *JAG* looking and feeling like a million bucks.

Although actors and actresses are in the business of looking good, *your* goals are just as important as any celebrity's. Whether your big role is as the bride or groom in your own wedding or you want to look your best for an anniversary, a high-school reunion, or a first date, my program will work for you. It is a formula, pure and simple. It works for my most high-profile movie-star clients, and it will work for you. Don't worry. I'll be with you every step of the way, paving the road that takes you to your destination—on time! My eating strategies and exercise plans are based on *you*—who you are, the body you have, what you like, how you live, and, most important, the time you have. I know you want to hear that this is going to be easy. Sorry. What I *can* say is that it's simple.

There won't be any starvation, suffering (well, maybe just a little), or unnecessary exhaustion. My programs are structured to produce results, not pain. Many people fail in their weight-loss attempts because their goals are unrealistic. Others don't succeed because their plans are either unfocused, too tough, or too time-consuming. I will help you create real-world goals that are reachable, with clear, measurable steps toward those goals. I will encourage you to stay focused, but you can also adjust your eating and exercise plans to ensure that they don't become too challenging or too easy.

And though some celebrity trainers assume that everyone has "Hollywood access"—to a state-of-the-art-gym and a full staff, including a nanny and a personal chef—and all the time in the world, I don't. I work with celebrities, but I also understand the real world. Hey, I live in it. I'm busy. I run my own business and I'm the mother of a rambunctious little boy. I do it all with no extra help (except from my fabulous husband, of course)—no nanny, no housekeeper, no chef. I've also had times in my life when I struggled with my own weight. Diagnosed as a teen with an underactive, partially working thyroid gland, I have been on thyroid medication most of my life. So all my life I've had to work hard to look good. It's been a challenge, but it's made me understand *you* all the better. I have designed my programs and this book with reality in mind. It is practical and user-friendly, created for people who are busy and may not like to exercise but do love to eat. I understand that time is short, distractions are everywhere, exercise can be a pain, and fast food is cheap, plentiful, and tempting. But you can make significant changes in the time you *do* have—whether it's several months or only two weeks—if you're willing to work for it.

You *will* get results, but you have to earn them. Motivation counts, and you need to put in effort and you need to plan. No matter how much or how little time you have, the formula is straightforward. The key is not to alter it. All I'm asking you to do is stick to the program.

>>> **Catherine's Story**

Because I'm an actress, I've always been in pretty good shape. When I got pregnant, I worked out and paid attention to what I ate during my pregnancy because I wanted to stay in shape and get back to work fast after the birth of my baby.

But after my daughter, Gemma, was born, I decided to really get serious. I had listened to so many negative comments from other mothers about how their bodies had changed—for the worse—after their babies. I made a decision that I wanted my body to look better after the baby than before. It was a little bit crazy, but I decided to put pressure on myself, to show the world I hadn't lost it yet. So I agreed to be on the cover of *Stuff* magazine—in a bikini! I had three months to get ready for the shoot.

> **❝ I made a decision that I wanted my body to look better after the baby than before. It was a little bit crazy, but I decided to put pressure on myself, to show the world I hadn't lost it yet. ❞**
> —CATHERINE

Gemma was several weeks old when I started on my eating program. I had about 15 pounds to drop, but the main goal was to lose body fat and get lean. Since I was nursing, Gina helped make sure that I was eating well, and that I was eating enough to feed my baby. We both wanted to be careful and safe. Everything was very regimented, with lots of lean protein and vegetables. I weighed everything—four ounces of this, a cup of that, five almonds—which was fine with me. I liked not having to think about anything. Right away, I felt great. I was dropping the weight and I had a lot of energy.

Because I'd had a C-section, I couldn't start exercising immediately. After six weeks, Gina did my first workout with me. My favorite thing was exercising with Gemma. I had a gym in my house, so I'd put her in one of those wraps and get on the Stair-Master. I loved having her close, and the motion would put her to sleep. It was very sweet for both of us. Gradually I worked up to exercising four or five days a week, and as I got closer to the shoot, I bumped it up even more. Sometimes I did two workouts a day, including boxing or kickboxing.

On the day of the shoot I felt great. I had lost the weight and gotten my body fat from 19.5 to 16 percent. It was a wonderful accomplishment.

Gemma is four now, and my life is very busy. Because of my work, I always keep my weight in a certain range and pay attention to my eating and exercise habits. So now I stick to Gina's maintenance plan. It's a good, moderate diet that I can handle. There are carbs, just less of the bad carbs. A couple of nights a week, I have spaghetti or pizza, and if I want a piece of cake every once in a while, that's fine. What's great is that if I have a photo shoot or a wedding or something, I know I can get back on a stricter plan and bounce right back. ‹‹‹

In the pages that follow are the techniques I've used over the years with my many clients, friends, and family members to help them achieve their weight-loss and fitness goals in the time frame they requested. You will find testimonials from many of the wonderful people I've worked with scattered throughout this book, describing how they felt on their individual plans and how the experience changed their way of thinking and their lives. Although my programs always work when they are followed, I quickly realized that it didn't really matter if the people doing them didn't have their heart and soul fully into the process. So before you and I dive into *your* deadline, I need your commitment right now that you are doing this of your own free will. That this deadline is important to you. And that you are willing to do what it takes to change your body and your health from this point on for the better. For the rest of your life.

In chapter 1, you will find out the top reasons for being overweight, why you may be unmotivated, and what to do to fix it. There are solutions to the problems that are keeping you from attaining your fitness goals. Look for the ten best ways to get started on an exercise regimen and stick to it!

Chapter 2 gives you facts on what weight loss is really about. You will learn why we gain weight, why it's so hard to lose it, and why body fat—not necessarily weight—is what makes us look bad. You'll even find out about how fat can be both our enemy and our ally. Want to learn how much fat you *should* have? I cover that, too, along with the top three reasons why you're *not* the biggest loser—that is, what you may be doing that's keeping the fat on and keeping you from losing weight. You will also get a sneak peek at what an effective "food formula" should look like and why the "one size fits all" type of eating plan doesn't work. I even throw in the three best-kept weight-loss secrets.

In chapter 3, I explain the connection between exercise and weight loss and discuss why the best fitness intentions sometimes fall by the wayside. You will find out what the best, most current methods of exercise are for maximizing calorie burning and, ultimately, fat loss. And you will determine where you stand with *your* current level of fitness so that you can choose the appropriate workouts in the deadline chapters.

Chapter 4 is where your work begins. You will pinpoint your own unique weight-loss and fitness goals with the help of a series of questions that look at your lifestyle and exercise and eating habits. You will also learn the differences between short-term and longer-term goals in order to choose the deadline that's right for you. I will teach you how to record your statistics, the measurements that will show your progress once you dig in and begin working toward a deadline.

The real fun begins in chapter 5, where you will be primed for success. This chapter will guide you through getting started. Here, I offer everything you need to go for your goal.

Chapters 6, 7, 8, and 9 are the deadline chapters. Each offers a different, complete program—Three Months, Two Months, One Month, and Two Weeks, respectively, plus a bonus One-Week emergency deadline plan in chapter 9. Once you select a program, depending on how much time you have and your preference for short-term versus long-term goals, you can really get started.

Finally, in chapter 10, I offer tips, advice, and suggestions on how to move from a deadline program to a long-term health and fitness program. In other words, your new deadline will be the rest of your life.

Now turn the page. You've got a deadline to meet!

1

>>>>

Inspiration, Perspiration, Dedication

The harder you work, the harder it is to surrender.

—*Coach Vince Lombardi*

My clients are generally highly motivated. Celebrities have everything to gain by looking their best. Looking good is part of the job description in Hollywood, and actors and other performers can miss out on parts, have a hard time getting through their stage performances, or even get fired if they show up on set looking overweight and out of shape. And the noncelebs I work with are also very inspired—sometimes desperate—to achieve specific goals by certain deadlines. Looking good on your wedding day, on a first date, or at a class reunion is important—as big a deal as a role is to a television or film star.

You cracked open this book, so I'm sure that you're motivated, too. But you might need an extra push, particularly after you've gotten started. I'm not going to lie to you. Sticking with any exercise and eating program, no matter how bad you want to lose weight and get in shape, is difficult, as anyone who's ever tried it knows—including me. You have to be ready—ready to work—and you have to want to achieve your goal. If you don't really *want* to lose 10 pounds or fit into that size 8 dress or walk into your twentieth-anniversary party looking fit and fabulous, then there's nothing I can say or do or teach you that is going to change that.

The definition of motivation is simple: "Having the desire and willingness to do something." In other words, it's on you. I'm not some psycho drill sergeant who's going to bark at you (in print!). You don't need that. This book is in your hands because you're a self-starter with a goal in mind. I'm your coach and your trainer and what I can do for you is offer specific, personalized tools that will make it easier for you to succeed. I will build your confidence by helping you create a program that's right for you and help you track your results so that you can see the progress you've made and be motivated by your success. What I will also do is remind you, from time to time, *Yes, you can! You really can.*

>>> Joanna's Story

Six months before my wedding, I needed to lose weight, so I reached out to Gina. I knew everybody would be looking at me, so it was the one day in my life that I wanted to look and feel my absolute best. I started way ahead of my wedding because I wanted to take my time and lose weight in a gradual way.

> 66 All of us learned how to change the way we ate for the rest of our lives, so that we can keep the weight off. 77
> —JOANNA

After doing all kinds of tests and assessments, Gina put me on a healthy diet composed of carbs, veggies, protein, and a little healthy fat. I cut out wheat and dairy after finding out I had an intolerance to them. Before that, I wasn't a junk-food addict; my problem was consistency. I'd munch on this and that throughout the day. But with the eating plan, I was able to focus. I also exercised five or six times a week, doing mainly cardio. By my wedding, I had lost 15 pounds.

Both of my parents decided they wanted to lose weight, too. My mother wasn't overweight, but she had been diagnosed with osteoporosis, and needed a plan to build her bones. Gina helped her change her eating habits and encouraged her to walk and do weight training. Though my mom had never exercised before, she ended up in the best shape of her life.

My father was a different story when he started. He is six foot one, weighed about 300 pounds, and had high cholesterol. We had been pushing him to lose weight, but the wedding got him motivated. He went on a healthy, protein-rich diet with no alcohol and no added table salt, and Gina got him to power walk. By the wedding, his weight loss was dramatic. He had lost 50 pounds in four months, and he's been able to keep it off.

At the wedding, I felt wonderful, and everyone was commenting on how great both my mom and dad looked. The reason it worked for us is that the approach is very reasonable. It's not at all extreme, and it makes sense. Plus, it's a lifetime plan. All of us learned how to change the way we eat for the rest of our lives, so that we can keep the weight off. <<<

Motivation—Just the Facts

Because I'm a numbers person, it has been important for me to understand inspiration, motivation, success, and failure from an intellectual standpoint. In other words, I like data, research, the facts. So I looked at the results of a survey of trainers and also conducted a study of my own to find out what makes some people stick to a plan, while others drop out or never get started. I was also interested to understand why people thought they were in the condition they were in. In other words, how had they reached a point where they needed me? I surveyed 800 women and men on my Web site and asked them, "Why do you think you are overweight and/or out of shape?" Here's what they said:

- 43%: Lack of motivation
- 42%: Laziness
- 5%: Lack of time
- 5%: Lack of exercise/bad eating habits
- 3%: Illness
- 2%: Pregnancy

Since lack of motivation was the number one reason people ended up out of shape and overweight, I decided to look closely at what caused people to lose motivation. From a survey of trainers, coaches, and other professionals who work with clients, here are the top seven reasons clients don't stick to the program:

1. They don't know what to do to get good results or are bored by the program.
2. They don't like working out.
3. They don't have the discipline to stick to it.
4. It's too expensive (gym memberships, home equipment, etc.).
5. They're too busy.
6. It's too hard (inconvenient) to get to the gym.
7. They've tried losing weight before and failed.

Finally, and most important, I looked at the positive—what *does* motivate someone to work out and eat well, or at least to begin making changes? Here's what respondents said:

- 44%: Someone's holding me accountable.
- 41%: I love feeling good.
- 10%: I've got a big event coming up.
- 4%: I don't like how I look or how clothes fit.
- 1%: My doctor said I had to.

Get Started, Stick to It: The Ten Best Ways

All right. So far, here's what we know. The best kind of program is interesting, varied, and somewhat fun; it is convenient, isn't too time-consuming, makes you feel good, shows your success, doesn't cost a lot and, finally, *works*. So with this knowledge plus what I know from working with thousands of clients, I have come up with ten tips for getting motivated and staying committed to an eating plan and an exercise program.

1. *Choose a realistic, reachable goal.* People kid themselves: we think we should be able to see dramatic results right away. Fitness books bank on unrealistic goals. "Lean, flat abs in just 30 seconds a day!" "Drop 10 pounds by June 1". . . but it's May 30! When you expect a result that's not humanly possible, you won't see success and you'll feel discouraged.

   Choosing a realistic goal increases motivation by allowing you to have a win. And that goal has to be *your* goal, specific to you and the way you live. Everybody and every *body* are not the same. For example, if you're muscular already, you might lose weight very quickly. But if you have a family history of obesity, it may take longer. So it's key to work toward a reachable goal for you. As soon as you begin to see results, you'll be pumped up and inspired to work even harder.

2. *Ask the hard question—what is ruining you?* How is this extra weight affecting your life? Then *use* that answer every single day to keep you moving toward your goal. So if your weight and physical condition are making your clothes too tight, keeping you from walking up the stairs without huffing and puffing, causing people to make fun of you, or getting in the way of your meeting your soul mate, think about these feelings when you don't want to work out or every time you want to eat something that isn't good for you. This will remind you why you got started in the first place and spur you to go on.

3. *Have a clear method for measuring your results.* Statistics don't lie, but people do. That's why I use numbers and graphs. I

look at pounds, of course, but I also take measurements, including body fat. So if the numbers have gone down, clearly the program is working. There's no gray area. Seeing results—in black and white—builds confidence and increases willpower.

4. *Make sure your program is tailored to your specific lifestyle.* Your eating plan and workout program have to be comfortable (well, at least for the most part), convenient, and easy on you; otherwise you'll want to skip and cheat. For instance, if you hit the snooze button five times in the morning and have to drag yourself out of bed, exercising in the a.m. isn't going to work for you. Instead, you'd do better working out at lunchtime and then eating afterward—or having a healthy snack around 4 p.m. and then exercising after work. Another way to make your program fit into the way you live is to adjust your current lifestyle to make room for exercising and eating right on a regular basis. So instead of getting out of bed and going straight to your computer to check your e-mail—and leaving no time to eat breakfast before running off to work—change things up. Eat breakfast first to get it out of the way, and then go to your computer. Or check your BlackBerry while you eat. The important thing is to make it work for *you*.

5. *Create small wins.* Come up with targets that are real to you and that you can accomplish in a reasonable amount of time. Like losing 1 to 3 pounds a week, or 2 inches from your waist in two months. Your targets don't have to focus on your body. You might aim for getting in 1 hour of exercise a day, or cutting out the calorie-rich coffee drink and replacing it with a nonfat cappuccino. These kinds of small wins add up and prevent you from feeling frustrated and wanting to quit.

6. *Reward yourself.* As you achieve your smaller targets and bigger goals, allow yourself a reward, like new clothes, a trip, jewelry, a movie, or whatever makes you feel good. (By the same token, if you miss your targets, abstain from any rewards or extra fun

until you have *earned* your way back.) The reward reinforces your success. Food, obviously, isn't the best reward.

7. *Keep the game fresh.* Have you ever seen people doing the same workout for years? I have. And they don't look any different. They seem almost robotic when you watch them. Change your routine periodically! It's best for you and best for your body. You get better results when you put new stresses—good stresses—on the body.

8. *Make adjustments when things aren't working.* If the routine, the time frame, and the meals you have chosen aren't fitting *you*, make adjustments so that they do. There is *always* a way to fix things and get on track. Believe me, I have seen and heard every problem, excuse, and disaster. And I have always found a way to make it work.

9. *Follow-up is key.* Keep track of your changes. Be aware of your weight, body fat, number of push-ups or other exercises you can do, and so on. If your goal is to change your measurements or lower your blood pressure, monitor these things. Make regular visits to your doctor if you are currently on medications for illnesses or conditions such as diabetes, high blood pressure, or thyroid disease. I have seen many people get off and stay off medications after getting on the right eating plan and exercise program. That should be motivation enough!

10. *Make good habits a habit.* The changes you make in the way you eat and exercise shouldn't be temporary, just to lose weight. Looking good, feeling healthy, and staying in shape is a lifelong process. Be sure that the changes you make *stay* in your daily routine and become your new habits. Once your new, healthy ways become routine, they feel comfortable. The easier you make things, the more you'll want to do them.

2

> > > >

The Food Formula

That whisper you keep hearing is the universe
trying to get your attention.

—*Oprah Winfrey*

Chances are you've tried to lose weight in the past but either
didn't succeed at all or lost some but weren't able to keep it
off. That's the case with most of the people I work with. So before we
get down to business and start knocking off your extra pounds—and
keeping them off for good—it's important to understand why you're
carrying around excess weight in the first place and why your
attempts to lose it haven't worked.

When you come right down to it, weight loss is really all about fat.
And I don't mean fat in your diet. I mean fat on your body. The first
thing my clients always say is "I need to lose weight; I'm too heavy."
But what they really mean is "I've got too much fat on my body."

Of course, fat isn't all bad. Our bodies need it in order to function.
We have a couple of different types of fat and each has an important
purpose. There is *essential fat* and *storage fat*. The storage fat is the

kind most people are concerned about. This fat is used as fuel for the body, but it is also the type that looks lumpy and ugly under the skin when we have too much of it. Essential fat surrounds our vital organs to protect them and is also used for immune system and hormonal function.

Unfortunately from an aesthetics point of view, women have more body fat than men—up to four times more. But it's for a good reason: we have sex-specific fat in the breasts, hips, thighs, and pelvic area for childbearing and other hormone function. But knowing that doesn't make it easier to accept the fat when it's visible on our butt, thighs, and hips.

>>> Susan's Story

A number of years ago I moved from New York to Los Angeles. Let me just say it—I hate LA. I was miserable and started gaining weight. I'm five feet two, and I climbed up to 179 pounds. Can you imagine? I came to California and got fat in a thin land.

Ideally, I wanted to be around 145, so to get the weight off, I tried every program out there—Weight Watchers, Jenny Craig, Diet Center. They all worked, but it didn't stick. Slowly, I would gain back the weight. The last diet I tried called for strict calorie counting. I wasn't eating much at all—maybe 900 calories per day—so I didn't understand why once I hit a low, I would start putting the weight back on.

Right away Gina asked me to tell her, in detail, what I ate. I explained that I would start with a skim latte at around 11:30 a.m., eat like a bird most of the day, and then use all of my calories at dinner. What Gina told me was a shock: "Your metabolism is shot," she said. "To lose weight, you need to eat more."

> 66 What Gina told me was a shock: 'To lose weight, you need to eat more.' 99
> —SUSAN

Gina said that because I was eating so little, my body was starving. It was holding on to every little bit of fat, which kept me from losing weight. Instead, I needed to eat more. This idea seemed so foreign and so wrong, but I listened anyway.

The following week, I went on a program of three meals a day and a snack or two. For each meal, I could choose a protein, a vegetable carb, a regular carb, like brown rice, and a fat. I could also earn carbs and treats by exercising. I worked out sometimes, but when things fell apart, I would stop. These were mostly new concepts, particularly the idea of "earning" food treats.

I stayed on the eating plan and walked and lifted weights for three months. In that time, I lost about 12 pounds, dropping to a size 10. I continue to eat three meals a day, plus two snacks. I walk five or six days a week—maybe not 3 miles because I'm sixty-three!—but I do get out there. For me, this program is now my lifestyle. ‹‹‹

Why You're Not the Biggest Loser

If you've tried to lose fat but haven't been as successful as you'd like, join the club. There are many, many reasons why people can't get rid of their stubborn fat. But the top causes—the ones I see over and over—are eating too much; eating too little (no, this isn't a typo!), usually by skipping meals; eating the wrong things; and not exercising enough or correctly. Since this chapter covers food, let's focus on the first three.

1. *Eating too much.* You're thinking, *Duh*, but it may be more complicated than you imagine. Most people are notoriously off base about how much they're eating, particularly at one sitting. Portions are often hard to determine, especially in these supersized times. Even people who are trying to do the right thing get it wrong and may be consuming more than they think.

   For instance, weight-loss programs describe one portion of protein as being about the size of your palm. But what if you're an average-size woman with really big hands? Also, consider thickness. It's one thing to eat a thin-sliced chicken breast the size of your palm and another to eat a palm-sized steak that's

4 inches thick. The bottom line is, if you are eating too much—more food than your body can possibly use—you will have extra fat.

2. *Eating too little.* What? That's right. Many people have failed at weight loss because they didn't eat enough. If you cut calories way back—below what you need to function—your body will kick into survival mode. It will try to hold on to storage fat because it's the perfect form of energy. It can be converted into blood sugar, for example, which the brain needs. But if your storage fat gets too low, the body will start to eat away at lean tissue—at first from the muscles, and, at worst, from organs like the heart—in order to save what little fat is left. So not only do you hang on to fat (read: weight), but you're also putting your body at serious risk. You lose muscle strength and disturb the body's long-term ability to burn more calories at rest. Even people who succeed in losing weight by indiscriminately cutting back on what they eat generally don't look great, especially if they aren't exercising. Thin and flabby isn't a good combination.

3. *Eating the wrong thing.* Some people cut back on how much they eat, but what they do eat isn't good for them. For example, many people have told me that they skip breakfast and then eat a big lunch. By 3 p.m., they're exhausted, looking for a quick energy fix. So in the late afternoon, they go for the proverbial "police officer" snack: coffee with milk and sugar and a donut.

   In science terms, here's what happens: the body responds to all that sugary, processed, low-fiber food by producing more insulin. The "insulin response" works this way: as blood-sugar levels increase, the body responds by releasing insulin. Insulin is the ultimate fat-storing hormone—a hormone that moves glucose (sugar) from the blood into the muscles and fat cells for storage. So even if you haven't eaten *that* much, what you did consume is stored as fat.

This kind of eating pattern is unhealthy since the food is low in fiber and generally deficient in nutrients. Plus, it's usually accompanied by a "crash." See, insulin is also called "the hunger hormone." Once it drops your blood sugar to its lowest, it causes cravings for more high-carb foods, and guess what? You eat more high-carb foods, you store more fat, and the cycle keeps repeating itself.

Go Ahead, Lose It!

So now we understand the bottom line: If you reduce body fat, you will lose weight. The big bonus is that you'll lose inches as well! For the record, I am *not* from the "one diet fits all" mentality. I am a firm believer that eating plans must consider individuality because there are so many factors involved in why some people lose weight and others don't. Having said that, there are some specific guidelines that seem to work very well with almost everybody. These are the basis for a good program. From there, you can tweak it to suit your individual needs.

So, what does the perfect food plan look like? It would have these seven things:

1. *The magic number of total daily calories for* you *to lose weight.* In chapter 5, I'll ask you to calculate how much you should be eating to lose fat. In a nutshell, it works this way:

    First, using an online calculator, you'll determine your basal metabolic rate (BMR). In English: how many calories you burn at rest. This is the daily caloric requirement to maintain your current weight. Second, you'll factor in exercise by calculating your total caloric requirement. Of course, you're not doing *nothing* all day. If you do exercise, the amount of calories you need to maintain your current weight will be higher—yeah! Finally, you'll come up with your magic number: adjusted total calories—how many calories you can eat in a day and lose weight and fat. For example, a thirty-year-old woman who is five feet four, weighs 150 lbs, and is moderately active can eat 1,586 calories per day and still lose.

Don't worry, we'll go over this again in more depth in chapter 5.

2. *The right amount of protein, carbohydrates, and fats in each meal.* This is different from the old-school method of "food combining"—which meant not eating certain foods, like meat and fruit, together at one meal. Eating the right combination of foods simply means eating meals containing a protein, a vegetable, a healthy carb, and fat. Eating this way will keep your blood-sugar and insulin levels in check to prevent fat storage.

3. *Meals every 2 to 4 hours consistently every day regardless of your old meal-skipping habits.* Consuming several small, balanced meals—plus a couple of snacks—keeps your blood-sugar levels even to prevent your body from storing fat. Plus, your energy level will stay up and you'll avoid the kinds of highs and crashes you may have gotten used to but which have been hurting you.

4. *No processed, junky foods loaded with refined sugar, hydrogenated oils, or trans fats.* Sugar is destructive. Period. Bad fats are destructive. Period. High amounts of sugar in the blood guarantees high insulin (hello, diabetes!), along with high triglycerides and cholesterol—all bad stuff.

5. *No alcohol.* Unless it's your twenty-fifth wedding anniversary or you finally received your PhD, cut out alcohol completely—at least for a while. It has almost twice the number of calories as protein and can cause carbohydrate cravings. Drinking makes weight loss much more difficult. Consuming hard liquor, like vodka or gin, slows the metabolism down for hours, and it also enhances fat storage. Ouch!

6. *Lots of water, instead of sodas (diet or otherwise) or other calorie-laden beverages.* You've heard this before, but it's worth saying again—you must consume eight glasses of water a day. Every-

body—even my three-year-old son—knows that the body is made primarily of water. The body needs it. Drinking lots of water allows the brain to function, the heart to beat, the lungs to work. Best of all, water aids the metabolic process, which allows your body to process food. So get in the habit of drinking water all the time.

7. *A commitment to change.* You'll need to make serious "lifestyle adjustments" since your current lifestyle isn't working for you. This is where Commitment with a capital C is critical. Your routines and habits have gotten you into the condition you're in now. It's time to Change (with a capital C).

What's So Bad About Diet Soda?

Stacks of research have linked drinking regular soda with obesity. But diet soda's not the answer either. New research has found that adults who drink regular soda (otherwise known as liquid candy) or diet soda have about a 50 percent higher risk of metabolic syndrome—a condition marked by high blood sugar, high blood pressure, high triglycerides, and obesity. All these double your risk for heart disease, stroke, and diabetes.

Another study, out of the University of Texas, noted that drinking even one *diet* soda a day increased the risk for being overweight by 41 percent. How? It may be that the sweet taste without the calories somehow affects the primitive appetite-control mechanism in our brains. This then triggers cravings and causes us to eat much more food. It's like we are searching for those "missing" calories. Plus, most diet sodas contain the artificial sweetener aspartame, which breaks down in the body to formaldehyde, a known poison. So, when it comes to soda, I listen to my friend and colleague Dr. Jonny Bowden: "Bottom line: soda's just about the worst drink possible—and that goes for both the regular and diet versions."

Stick to water. Even if you aren't on a fat-loss program, you should still be drinking at *least* 64 ounces of water a day to maintain a normal healthy metabolism. If you have trouble getting enough, try keeping a 32-ounce bottle with you that you can refill. Put one in your car, office, gym bag, hotel room; take one on the airplane, to a business meeting, or social gathering and to every other possible event or place that I didn't mention. It should be a part of you wherever you go. Always. The best kind of water is either distilled or purified. However, some municipal water in this country is so good that we don't ever really need to import another bottle from France, Italy, or some obscure island.

Any Questions?

Regardless of the deadlines my clients are working toward, I'm often asked a number of questions about what to eat and what not to eat while on my program. Here are answers to some common concerns:

What if I get tired when I'm on one of the stricter-deadline programs and don't have energy to exercise?

Although you shouldn't, if you happen to feel a little less energetic from the new changes in your eating plan, try having a meal 40 to 60 minutes before your workout.

I've been told that when I'm dieting I should eliminate wheat, dairy, and sugar. Is this true?

Maybe. Wheat, dairy, and sugar may slow down weight loss for *some* people. Many nutritionists and holistic professionals recommend that you eliminate these foods if you are particularly sensitive to them—some people are even allergic. Not to mention that nonorganic dairy products are loaded with antibiotics, hormones, and other drugs used to keep the cows healthy and fat. Yes, fat! If you choose to eat dairy, go for the raw or organic types. If you feel your weight loss is slower than what is expected on your deadline plan, consider eliminating these products one at a time.

What's the deal with artificial sweeteners?

To me, this falls into the category of religion and politics. Some nutritionists are completely against all artificial sweeteners and others are okay with certain ones. Here's my take on them based on the information we have available to us today.

Equal (aspartame)—*One thumb up, one thumb down.* The FDA has reported side effects like seizures, dizziness, increased liver enzymes, visual impairment; however . . . many people never experience these symptoms.

Splenda (sucralose) and Sweet'N Low (saccharin)—*Two thumbs up.* Splenda has the best reports to date. Sweet'N Low, although banned many years ago when it was associated with cancer, has since been put back on the safe list. The link to cancer showed up in research conducted on rats—which ingested enough to saccharin to equal eight hundred cans of diet soda a day. No wonder they developed tumors!

Stevia—*Two thumbs up*. This is an herb that has a definitive aftertaste. Other than that it seems pretty safe.

Sugar Twin (cyclamates)—*One thumb up, one thumb down*. This has caused cancer in rats, but is still on the safe list. Most nutritionists feel that in small amounts it may be okay.

Can I eat protein bars on any of the deadline programs?

Well . . . no. Protein bars seem innocent when it comes to carbs, but many of the labels are misleading. Often they say something like "only 2 grams of usable carbs." What does that mean? It refers to sugar alcohols that don't have the same effect on blood sugar as other carbs do. But they're still carbs. Once you move to your maintenance program, you can have bars periodically. But until then, steer clear.

Are protein-powder shakes allowed on the deadline programs?

Absolutely! In fact, they are a great source of protein when you are tired of eating fish, chicken, and turkey. They're also quick and easy to make and take with you. I travel a lot, and taking protein powder in small bags has saved me numerous times when there was not much else available. But avoid shakes labeled "meal replacements." Protein powders are *all* protein with no other ingredients. Meal-replacement shakes have protein, carbs (often in the form of sugar), and fat. Stick with the pure protein powders.

What about fish—are some better than others?

Yes. My weight-loss plans call for a moderate amount of protein, so if you don't eat meat—and even if you do—fish is a great choice. These fish choices are higher in omega-3 fatty acids and low in contaminants:

- Abalone
- Anchovies
- Bay scallops
- Clams (U.S.)
- Crab
- Herring (Atlantic)
- Mackerel (Atlantic)
- Northern Canadian shrimp
- Oregon pink shrimp
- Oysters
- Pacific halibut (Alaskan)
- Sablefish/black cod (Alaskan)
- Sardines
- Shrimp
- Striped bass
- Tilapia (U.S.)
- Wild salmon (Alaskan)

These fish choices are not as healthy. They are higher in mercury or other contaminants:

- Atlantic salmon
- Bluefin tuna
- Caviar
- Chilean sea bass
- Grouper
- Marlin
- Orange roughy
- Rockfish
- Shark
- Swordfish
- Tilefish
- Wild sturgeon

Are all vegetables allowed on your eating plan?

Temporarily, no. Avoid these starchy vegetables until you reach your fat-loss goal:

- Beets
- Carrots
- Corn
- Parsnips
- Peas
- Plantains
- White potatoes
- Winter squashes (acorn and butternut)

SHHH: The Best-Kept Weight-Loss Secrets

Here are three weight-loss tips you might not have thought of:

1. Get plenty of sleep. I often notice that people who don't get enough sleep have trouble losing weight. Here's the reason: stress makes you fatter! You've heard of cortisol? It triggers insulin secretion and can cause insulin resistance. It breaks down muscle tissue and reduces your metabolic rate. And if that isn't enough, stress causes you to store fat around your middle, of all places! So be sure to get the good solid 7 to 8 hours of sleep experts recommend.

2. Consume lots of fiber. Fiber is the best-kept secret in weight loss. When you eat plenty of high-fiber foods like vegetables, whole grains, and whole wheat, instead of starchy carbohydrates and white rice, you can achieve great weight-loss results. Fiber helps speed up the movement of food through the digestive system. Some fiber doesn't get digested at all, so as it moves through the system, it cleanses the intestines, taking calories along with some fat and carbs with it. In fact, if you did nothing except add fiber to your diet, you would get *some* weight loss.

3. Timing is everything! Eat the right food at the right time. One of the best examples of eating the wrong thing at the wrong time would be eating cereal late at night. Even if it's nonfat milk and Cheerios, the insulin response you will get from this combination will make you fatter. It is a misconception that milk is a high-protein food. Look at the label; it has just as many carbs as protein, or even more. On the other hand, if you were to consume a protein shake along with it or some hard-boiled egg whites, it would be an entirely different metabolic story. Another example of bad timing is eating fruit all by its lonesome. You can guarantee a fatter body if you do this. But if you add some light string cheese or some turkey slices, you will not get the same response. Get the idea?

Is it okay to use cooking sprays when preparing food?

Yes! In fact, it's the best way to cut unwanted fat and calories that come from using butter, oils, and margarine.

What about salad dressing sprays instead of salad dressing?

An excellent choice! Salad sprays taste great, and ten sprays contain about 1 gram of fat, 1 gram of carbs, and only 10 calories. Pay attention to sodium, though: 100 milligrams per ten sprays. Still, not bad!

Now you know why you may have had trouble losing weight in the past and the basics about how to get rid of it. In the coming chapters, I will ask you to collect lots of very specific data, and you will use this information to design a personalized food plan. You will also find tips and tricks on how to handle situations when you are traveling, at social events, or simply do not have certain things available to you to eat for whatever reason. But remember, we have a deadline to meet, so let's move on to the exercise section of the program.

3

> > > >

The Exercise Equation

Do it.
Do it right.
Do it right now.

—*NASA slogan*

Whether you have six months or six days, without a doubt, you can lose weight just by adopting a smarter, healthier way of eating. However, without exercise, your body will be thin but flabby, and your metabolism will be sluggish. Adding cardiovascular, strength, and flexibility training into the mix will get you toned and tightened and rev up your metabolism to speed weight loss and keep off the pounds. It doesn't have to take a lot of time, either. I'm all for working efficiently. But the one thing I do ask of you is that you train hard . . . at whatever level you fit into at the time. Believe me, you don't get results from days, weeks, and months of namby-pamby workouts.

Without strength training to develop muscles and the heart-pumping element to help shed fat, you're not going to get results—period. But let's face it, you don't have time to work out for several hours a day; that would be like having another full-time job.

One of my best-kept secrets (although no secret to my many successful colleagues) is to combine strength training and cardiovascular exercise to minimize your workout time but maximize your results. There are many different ways to train both energy systems at the same time. For example, *circuit training*. As you move through a series of light resistance exercises and cardio stations, or "circuits," you keep your heart rate up while increasing muscle tone. *Peripheral Heart Action* (PHA) *training* is similar to circuit training but even

How Hard Are You Working?

How do you know if your workout is effective? Are you getting a good workout or coasting, barely breaking a sweat? Use these four ways to gauge cardio intensity:

1. **Wear a Heart Rate Monitor.** This is the simplest, most effective way to measure cardio training. You can monitor your heart rate at any given moment of your workout without stopping by wearing the chest strap and watch or any of the various styles of heart monitors. There is even a new heart rate ring available from Lifespan Fitness that fits on your finger, and most cardio machines now have built-in heart-rate monitors.

2. **Determine Your Training Heart Rate.** Turn to the end of chapter 4 and read the section on training heart rate. You can calculate it by going to the tools and calculators section of my Web site, www.ginalombardi.com.

3. **Monitor Your Rate of Perceived Exertion.** Your Rate of Perceived Exertion is how hard you *feel* you're working out; how hard you're breathing. On a scale of 1 to 10, 10 means you're at your max, while 1 is easiest. Aim for an intensity of 3 to 5 if you are a beginner and 4 to 7 as you progress to ensure a good workout.

Minimum

0	Nothing at all
0.5	Very, very weak
1	Very weak
2	Weak
3	Moderate
4	Somewhat strong
5	Strong
6	
7	Very strong
8	
9	
10	Very, very strong

Maximum

4. **Use a Pedometer.** This inexpensive little gadget senses movement and can tell you how many steps you've taken, whether you're treadmill walking, jogging outside, stair-climbing, or cleaning the house. Every time you take a step, it gets counted. Look at how many steps you're taking in a one-minute period. The more you take, the harder you're working. A pedometer can also track the distance you've traveled and estimate how many calories you've burned.

tougher since it involves heavier weights. The exercises are strategically ordered, with lower body followed by upper body, followed by lower body, et cetera. This adds a tremendous cardiovascular effect. Both of these workouts are multipurpose and result in faster benefits in less time than doing weights and cardio separately.

>>> **Deirdre's Story**

When I was in my mid-thirties, my life was very, very hectic. I'm in real estate development, and I was working too much, traveling too much, and sitting on my ass too much. One day I looked up and I was about 30 pounds overweight. I was also tired all the time. When I received a brochure in the mail from Gina, I knew I was ready to turn that around. I looked at her picture on the brochure and decided I wanted to look like her.

Right away I learned that in order to lose weight, I needed a total approach—eating and exercise. Nutrition was the easier part. First Gina dispelled a lot of myths I had picked up from talking to friends and reading diet-related articles in newspapers and magazines. I thought it was okay to not eat all day and then consume a day's worth of calories at dinner. Wrong. Gina taught me the importance of eating smaller, balanced meals throughout the day and the value of protein in the diet.

> **Even after I met my goal and went from feeling pudgy, sluggish, and tired to being a hot little mama, I still loved exercise—which was a big deal for a couch potato who hadn't done anything for twenty years.**
> —DEIRDRE

Exercise was a bigger problem. I had an aversion to working out. My history with exercise was hiding in the back row in gym class. Fitness required effort and perspiration, and those were two things I preferred to avoid in favor of watching movies and munching on popcorn.

But Gina explained the importance of exercising and started me out walking three times a week, both on the treadmill and up and down the hills in my neighborhood. In a short time, I realized that what people said about exercise was true: I felt much better and had more energy. Overall I felt more alive. Soon I added strength training to my cardio workout. I worked out with an exercise ball, lifted weights. After a couple of weeks, with the eating but especially because of the strength training and cardio, I saw the results in my body. In four and a half months, I lost 40 pounds.

Even after I met my goal and went from feeling pudgy, sluggish, and tired to being a hot little mama, I still loved exercise—which was a big deal for a couch potato who hadn't done anything for twenty years. ⟪⟪⟪

I Know I Should Exercise, But . . .

In my business I hear a lot of "buts." Of course, many of these excuses are valid. However, if you want to get in shape, feel good in body *and* mind, and lose weight, you've got to work out. And if you choose your exercises wisely, and do them correctly, you'll have fun and feel great. So let's have a conversation:

I would exercise, but . . .

You: "I'm too busy."

Me: "What you've been 'busy' doing is making you fat! Change your work schedule, get up earlier, come home later. Do what you have to do to make it work. Redesign your life so that it works *for* you, not *against* you."

You: "I hate going to the gym."

Me: "Well, there's the obvious solution, which is to work out at home or get a gym buddy to help distract you from your hatred of the gym. But the more important and less obvious solution is to change up your routine. There are countless exercises and variations of these exercises to make your workouts fun, challenging, and motivating. Once you start having a good time, it won't matter where you're working out; you'll want to do it."

You: "It's boring."

Me: "Trust me, you could *never* do the same workout until the end of time. By changing the number of sets and reps, the order of exercises, the equipment used—or maybe just using body weight, or even doing exercises according to seconds or minutes instead of reps, for example—you will experience a different feeling every time you train. *This* is the key to staving off boredom. And if you happen to be interested in an activity like bowling or a sport like basketball or softball, you can tailor your workouts to make you better at those games. You can also change your environment by exercising outdoors, like at the beach, in the mountains, or at a park."

You: "I'm too tired."

Me: "Assess *why* you're tired. If it's because you're not getting enough sleep, get some. If it's because you're sitting at a desk all day—I don't buy it. You may be mentally fatigued, but your body has plenty of energy. Try doing your workout first thing in the morning and you'll feel energetic all day. Commit to it for two weeks and see what happens. You won't remember what it felt like to be tired."

You: "I'm too fat to exercise."

Me: "Nice try. Even if you're a hundred pounds overweight, you have to start somewhere. Walking should be your primary focus as well as sticking to a solid eating plan."

You: "I don't know what I'm doing."

Me: "Playing dumb may work for you in other areas of life. On the other hand, this can be a valid point. But this book gives you the guidelines to do the right thing, so no more excuses!"

What Went Wrong?

If you're like many of the people who have come to me, you may have started an exercise program but became frustrated when you didn't lose weight—or didn't lose it fast enough. Not seeing results quickly may have gotten the best of you, and you dropped out. What did you do wrong? Let's take a good look so that it never happens to you again.

Fitness Primer

Fitness isn't rocket science, but there is some jargon you should know. Learn the words on this list so you can understand the lingo once you choose a deadline and start your workouts.

Duration. The amount of time you spend on the exercise. For cardio this is measured in minutes; for resistance training, in reps or seconds performing an exercise. The duration will depend on the workout you choose.

Exercise or Cardio Mode. The actual resistance (weight-training) exercises or type of cardio (treadmill, stair-climbing, etc.) you will be doing.

Frequency. How many times per week you will need to do the exercises. Every workout program specifies the number of days you will work out.

Intensity. How hard you should be working; for resistance training it would be in sets, reps, and weight. For cardio it would be either Rate of Perceived Exertion (see the chart on page 30) or heart-rate range (see the formula for calculating heart-rate range on page 53).

Intervals. *Interval training* is the technique of incorporating several short bursts of high-intensity exercise followed by longer active recovery periods in one training session. The result is more total calories burned and a faster increase in cardiovascular fitness.

Progression. In order to change your body, you will have to change up your exercise program periodically. Progression is a very important part of getting fit. Increasing weights, intensity (sets/reps/heart rate), or length/type of cardio training will help you progress.

Here's what an interval workout looks like:

After warming up, perform 30 seconds of exercise at a high intensity followed by 2 minutes at a low to moderate intensity as directed below. Refer to chapter 4 to figure out your heart-rate maximum (HR max) or go to my online calculator at www.ginalombardi.com.

Example

5-minute warm-up

30 seconds at 80 to 85 percent HR max

2 minutes at 55 to 75 percent HR max

30 seconds at 80 to 85 percent HR max

2 minutes at 55 to 75 percent HR max

30 seconds at 80 to 85 percent HR max

2 minutes at 55 to 75 percent HR max

30 seconds at 80 to 85 percent HR max

2 minutes at 55 to 75 percent HR max

30 seconds at 80 to 85 percent HR max

2 minutes at 55 to 75 percent HR max

30 seconds at 80 to 85 percent HR max

2 minutes at 55 to 75 percent HR max

5-minute cooldown

Maybe you are the person who gets gung-ho about starting an exercise program and hits it hard for a month or two and then the gym membership card slips to the back of your wallet and eventually gets removed and retired to a drawer in your desk. Or are you the one who goes to the gym day in and day out, week in and week out, but still looks the same? Do you try every class known to man- and womankind only to find yourself exhausted from running around town and hundreds of dollars poorer to boot? Do you find yourself wanting to change your body, your bad habits, your life, but just don't know how to do it or where to start?

Do you feel that you are so far gone and out of shape that you are embarrassed to walk into a gym or even ask for help? Have you bought every product ever advertised in a television infomercial only to find that they really don't hang clothes that well?

If you are nodding your head "yes" to any or possibly *all* of these questions, I understand. Why? Because I have met every single one of you (at least once). There are only so many reasons why a human being is out of shape and stays that way. It's really not an unsolved mystery. So let me take your hand and lead you to the land of success.

What Kind of Shape Are You In?

It's important to know your current fitness level. There are basically three levels, with a lot of gray area in between. So read on to figure out which category is *generally* you.

Beginner. You're a beginner if you haven't formally exercised or been on a structured exercise program *ever* or in more than a year. So many times I have heard someone who is 50 pounds above her or his ideal weight say, "I'm going to start running to get in shape," but she or he isn't conditioned enough to begin running. You don't run to get in shape. You get in shape to be *able* to run. Running is a tough exercise even for someone who *is* in shape. So starting off with it is fitness suicide. If you're out of shape, I ask that you exercise every other day and then add on from there. Otherwise, you'll burn out. On the nonexercise days, focus on improving your eating habits, getting organized, and getting your life in order so that this condition will never come back to haunt you.

Intermediate. I'd call you an intermediate exerciser if you've been pretty consistent at working out at the gym or involving yourself in sports activities at least three times a week for a year or more. Right after you work out you feel really good, but later you're tired and you feel as if three times a week or so is all you can handle. You might also be working out more than three times a week but not getting results anymore. A change in your program and regular tune-ups are all you need.

Advanced. You're an advanced exerciser if you do a good amount of exercise, maybe even work out on a daily basis, with an occasional "slow period" where you cut back for a few weeks and then pick it up again. You may have hit a plateau in terms of strength, weight loss, or body-fat loss even though you are training at a higher level than most. If fat loss is your goal, your eating habits and/or the way you are structuring your workouts may be keeping you from reaching your goals. It may also be that your eating habits aren't as good as you thought. We can handle that, too.

Note: Although this book is more for the beginner and intermediate level exerciser, I do have bonus sections with advanced programs.

Free Weights or Machines?

In my weight-training program, I ask you to use free weights. However, you may prefer machines, either at home or at the gym. So in each deadline program, I've included machine workouts.

Choosing between free weights and machines is really quite simple. Use what you feel more comfortable with and/or what's in your budget and what's readily available to you, whether you're at the gym, at home, or traveling. But keep the pros and cons on page 37 in mind if you have specific needs:

Free weights

Advantages	Disadvantages
Require other muscles to come into play, specifically stabilizer muscles, giving you more bang for the buck	Don't compensate for the "easier" portion of the motion, like at the top, or "lock out," of a bench press, for example
Do not limit you to a specific range of motion	Sometimes you may need a limited or fixed range of motion if you have an injury
Can mimic everyday movements as well as sport-specific movements	May require more control and skill to maneuver than machines
Do not limit you to the single function of a machine	
Portable and affordable	

Machines (Resistance Machines, Cable Systems, Rubber Tubing)

Advantages	Disadvantages
Are designed to compensate for the "easier" portion of the movement by increasing resistance at that point in the exercise	Tend to isolate muscles and therefore do not bring other muscles into play to assist or stabilize
Some companies, like Nautilus, have made specific machines just for women and smaller-framed exercisers	Most machines do not always fit the person who is using them (for example, if you're tall, short, or obese, or even have a small skeletal frame, machines will not accommodate your individual needs)
Some people feel more comfortable in a fixed position	Many people are more likely to get injured on machines because they feel they are "safer" and don't pay as close attention to what they are doing
Some cable machines (like FreeMotion) and rubber tubing *can* mimic everyday "functional" movements and athletic movements	Most machines isolate a muscle or a muscle group in a fixed range of motion and do *not* mimic functional movements
	Machines are *very* expensive for home purchase

Here's a question a lot of people ask me: Do you burn more calories using an elliptical trainer or a treadmill?

Though the elliptical trainer may seem easier, the answer is you get a similar benefit from both. According to a study published in the *Journal of Sports Medicine and Physical Fitness*, 22 moderately active women participated in a twelve-week aerobic training program consisting of three sessions per week on a treadmill or an elliptical trainer. They worked out very hard for over an hour. Surprisingly, everybody, regardless of which machine they used, burned about the same amount of calories and got a similar cardiovascular boost.

With that in mind, the more important question is how do you get the best workout? Here's the secret: on either of those machines, do interval training—speed up your pace for 30 to 60 seconds and take it back down for 30 to 60 seconds and repeat for 30 to 40 minutes. Doing "intervals" will not only burn more *total* calories—including fat calories—per workout, but will also increase the amount of postexercise calories you burn. Use a machine that adds in arm/upper-body work and you can increase calorie burning by even more . . . as long as you don't ease up on your legs once you start working your arms.

One more important point: the elliptical machine is easier on the body than the treadmill, so it's a better choice if you're carrying a lot of extra weight or have lower-back, knee, or other lower-body joint problems. The key to success on either machine if you want to burn the most calories is to train smart but hard. And remember, the harder you train, the more postexercise burn you'll get!

Gain, No Pain!

It's great to train hard, but important to do it with care to avoid injury. No matter what level of fitness you're at right now, there are a few things to always keep in mind when you're working out:

Get good at identifying the difference between "pain," "muscle fatigue," and "injury." If you're feeling sharp *pains* during an exercise, *stop* and get checked out by a doctor. If you feel as if you've *injured* something (a muscle, a tendon, a ligament, or a bone), *stop* what you're doing and see a physician right away. If you're feeling *muscle fatigue*, good job! You're working hard. Your muscles are building up waste products that cause the "burn." Take rest periods between exercises and be sure to drink water.

Don't do too much too soon. I know you want to get there fast, but overdoing it right out of the gate could get you knocked out of the game for a while. So end your workouts feeling good about what you did—not too much, not too little, and wanting more!

Always, always, always maintain proper form on every exercise, including cardio, and especially weight training. Be sure to keep your neck and back in alignment and your wrists aligned with your arms. Your knees and elbows should always be in a "soft" position; don't overextend or "lock" them, since this can be very damaging over time to the joints and the surrounding tissue. When on cardio machines, stand upright and don't lean on . . . well . . . anything!

Even if you're short on time, always warm up for 5 to 10 minutes before weight training or cardio exercises. Do light treadmill or outdoor walking, cycling, stair-climbing, or even the old-school standards, jumping jacks or jogging in place. Stretch lightly only after your warm-up. Stretching *is not* a warm-up, contrary to what your grammar-school coach may have told you. In fact, many studies have shown that too much stretching prior to athletic activities can actually decrease performance and, in some cases, cause injury. Save your serious stretching for the end of the workout.

Got it? Good. No more excuses. Let's get down to business. You're one step closer to that deadline.

4

Go for the Goal

A goal is a dream with a deadline.

—*Napoleon Hill*

Before you design the eating plan and exercise program that works for you, we need to figure out how much weight you'd like to lose, how much time you have, what you like to eat, which kinds of exercise you enjoy most, and what your schedule is really like. In this chapter, we will come up with a goal that's right for you.

Most people come to me with unrealistic expectations. This is pretty typical: "I need to lose fifteen pounds in two weeks for a TV show" or "I need to lose ten pounds by Saturday" (and it's Monday). Is it *possible* to do this? Maybe. Is it safe and long-lasting? No. The trick is to know what the body, *your* body, is capable of in the amount of time you have and then work with it—not against it—to achieve that goal. So then the question is, what *is* realistic?

Most people can expect to see up to a 10-pound weight loss in two weeks. Notice I said "up to," because everyone responds differently to changes made to his or her usual eating habits and exercise program (or lack thereof). So this kind of result means committing to a strict eating plan, not a starvation plan, and a reasonable amount of exercise. Your results will match both the effort you put in and your body's response. It's also important to remember that although the scale will tell you one thing—how many pounds you've lost—your body is changing in other ways, too. For example, losing 6 pounds in two weeks may not seem like a big deal to you, but you may have also dropped 2 inches from your waist and reduced your body fat. Those are great results!

What's Your Goal?

To come up with a realistic goal, start by answering these two questions:

1. *Why* do you want to lose this weight and get into shape?
2. How is your current condition "ruining" your life?

(Examples: "I don't fit into my clothes anymore, and it's frustrating"; "I am forty, recently divorced, and getting back into the dating game, and I don't feel good about myself"; "I am too young to be this overweight; it makes me depressed and self-conscious, and people make fun of me.")

Whatever the reasons, they are real to *you*, and that's all that matters. Your answers to these questions are the driving force behind your commitment to stay loyal to this program and continue on it long after you've reached your ideal weight. They will be the reason you drag yourself out of bed in the morning and walk by the fridge without opening the door. Post your answers anywhere and everywhere you will see them. On your bathroom mirror, on your computer screen, on the refrigerator door, on the dashboard in your car. They will be a constant reminder of why you bought this book.

Next questions:

1. How much weight do you want to lose?
2. What's your deadline?

Remember to be realistic! Consider how much it is *possible* to lose and how much effort and time you're willing to put into that goal.

Short-Term versus Long-Term Goals

Short-term goals—those you want to achieve in a few weeks—are different from long-term goals, which you have several months to reach. Even if you have all the time in the world, you may choose a short-term goal because you like the intensity. Having a deadline motivates you. On the other hand, you may prefer a long-term goal because gradual changes are easier and less stressful. Making drastic changes can be too difficult mentally and physically for some, while others really embrace the challenge. Only you know you. Don't put yourself in a position to fail—perhaps again—by trying to do something you don't feel you can do.

My other philosophy on this goal issue is that many of us need a test in discipline. A good friend once told me that the quality of your life depends on how you react to things. If making strict changes in your lifestyle is what you need to get yourself in gear and reverse your downward spiral, go for the short-term goal and level out with a longer-term goal. If you have the luxury to choose, here are the pros and cons of each:

Quick and Dirty: Two to four weeks

The Pros: You'll get the jump start of your life! Seeing results quickly can be all you need to feel good about yourself again *and* stay on the path to a better body.

The Cons: It's strict and requires extreme discipline, which you may or may not have. There is virtually no room for slipups on a short-term program if you want to reap the full reward.

The Bottom Line: You shouldn't think of a short-term goal as a quick-fix program that you can do for a couple of weeks and then go back to your old ways. Instead, think short-term program, long-term results. If you choose a shorter program, after you've met your deadline, move over to my longer-term or maintenance program and be careful not to fall back into bad habits. In fact, promise me that you will not quit when those two or four weeks are up.

>>> Brenda's Story

I wanted to lose 8 to 10 pounds before my class reunion. The prospect of seeing old friends whom I'd been out of touch with for fifteen years was scary. I was desperate to walk into that room feeling like a million bucks in my little black dress. But I couldn't do that at five foot six and 144 pounds. I have two children and had not been able to get this weight off for eight years, and then I met Gina.

Right away, I learned that I had to get rid of my worst habit: skipping meals and going long periods without eating, then eating as much as humanly possible late at night. That was a habit I had gotten into because of my hectic work schedule and also being a mom.

> 66 I lost 9 pounds of fat in thirteen days and dropped nearly 2 inches from my waist. That postpregnancy pooch was virtually gone. 99
> —BRENDA

With a strict but definitely adequate eating plan and a walking program, I lost 9 pounds of fat in thirteen days and dropped nearly 2 inches from my waist. That postpregnancy pooch was virtually gone. Eating lean protein and fresh vegetables at each meal and cutting out dessert gave me energy like I had never had before and I felt full . . . unlike on other eating programs I have tried. At first I missed my sweets, but after seeing the results in just a couple of days, it was no task to stick with the plan. I was ecstatic. It made me want to stick to the program after my event, just to see if I could get 3 or 4 more pounds off and feel as if I had room to enjoy life.

But more important, it opened my eyes to how I was eating before and how far off target I was on a daily basis. My busy work and family schedule got me into terrible eating habits that were actually making me fat and keeping me fat. I'll never go back there again! If it wasn't for that short-term goal, I might not have had a reason to get myself going! <<<

The Longer Haul: Two to four months—or more

The Pros: Sometimes it's comforting to know that you're on a program that is flexible and a little more forgiving when it comes to time. When I write articles, it can be very stressful when my editor gives me an assignment and then tells me it's due the next day or in a couple of days. If I knew I had two months to do it, I could spend a little time getting used to the idea. Well, it's the same thing here. You may do better knowing that making smaller changes each day, each week, each month, will safely but surely get you to your goal. Minus the pressure.

The Cons: There really isn't a downside to taking the longer path. In fact, it's often a better choice. Lifestyle changes don't usually happen overnight. By taking three or four months to reach a reasonable goal, you can almost guarantee that you will not only get the weight off but also keep it off.

The Bottom Line: If you have the time, longer-term goals are a great way to go. Give yourself the opportunity to enjoy the gratification you'll feel when you take control of your life and your body. As you make the changes in your daily schedule to exercise, to eat right, to take better care of yourself, you are less likely to fall back into old patterns.

>>> Jack's Story

Little by little, my weight had crept up to 230 pounds. I wasn't in a *big* hurry, but I knew I needed to lose the excess weight when I could see that my waist was bigger than my chest. It's strange when you can't button your suit jacket anymore and have to go to meetings with the buttons undone all day. Also, I had been diagnosed with type 2 diabetes. I had never before had any health problems, and this scared me.

Over the years, I had developed some terrible eating habits. Always feeling rushed in the morning, I would skip breakfast and drink only black coffee. Sometimes I would even skip lunch. But then I would graze on nuts and raisins all day, not realizing that I was packing in the calories. At night, I'd come home, bone tired, and sit on the couch in front of the TV and eat lots of ice cream, or chocolates that were in the "for guests only" bowl on the coffee table. And to top it all off, I would lift weights maybe once a week or walk on the treadmill for 20 minutes if I was feeling guilty. All this of course brought me no results. I really needed to change.

I am not one who works well with the "cold-turkey" method. So I chose a program with a goal of 20 pounds in four to six months, because I felt that would be a comfortable, realistic time frame for me. My plan was gradual. Rather than removing lots of things from my diet, Gina added things that were healthier. For example, I started eating breakfast and realized that I actually like turkey bacon and egg whites wrapped up in a tortilla. And I instantly felt more energetic, because I was starting the day right. It also kept me from grazing on snack foods all day to make up for skipped meals.

> " I am not one who works well with the 'cold-turkey' method. So I chose a program with a goal of 20 pounds in four to six months. Much to my surprise, I lost 24 pounds in four months! "
> —JACK

Much to my surprise, I lost 24 pounds in four months! More than my actual goal! My waist went from 46 inches to 41¾ inches. My blood sugar stabilized, and that meant I could reduce my medication. A month later, I was off the diabetes medication completely.

I learned a lot from all this and will never really look at food the way I used to. I now realize that food is a necessity for survival, but used the wrong way, it can kill you! Having a four-month goal worked so well for me because I could get used to the changes and really make them stick. «««

By the Numbers

I'm a numbers person . . . to a point. When I'm working with someone, I pay close attention to statistics—weight, body fat, body circumferences, and blood pressure, as well as cholesterol and blood-sugar levels. Numbers are important at this stage of the game. Statistics are a great motivational tool, allowing you to track your progress and keep yourself in check on a weekly basis. Up until now, what you've been doing has been unsuccessful. We are going to change that. Eventually, you'll be able to lose the graphs and charts and just *know* that you are feeling and looking great without having to get on the scale anymore. This means that you have officially made a *lifestyle* change and arrived at the place where you are in control of your body! This is a happy day for you and for me.

Right away, you'll need to take all your "before" measurements. Although this isn't so fun for some, I insist on it. Sometimes people are not honest about what they're really doing each day. So when the time comes to compare numbers from four weeks ago to those from today, I *know* the numbers don't lie.

Your numbers will give you a starting point as well as a kick in the pants. They tell us where you are and point you to where you need to go. And then you'll need to keep measuring. Once you start moving toward a reachable goal, one that can be measured by watching as your stats begin to change, you'll see your goal getting closer. This success will spur you to continue working—and work harder.

So let's get to the data gathering right now.

Know the Score

This score sheet will be like your report card. Only this time, *you* are tracking the grades instead of the teacher. Take your measurements properly and carefully, as described in this section, so that your numbers will always be as accurate as possible. This score sheet is what will prove to you that your effort is being rewarded. After your initial measurements have been recorded, you will start your eating and exercise program. Then you will retest yourself four weeks from your start date. If you have a two-week goal, you can retest at the end of the two weeks. Then change over to your longer-term program and begin retesting every four weeks.

Score Sheet

Name: _____

Start Date: _____
Deadline Date: _____

BODY MEASUREMENTS

Date: _____   Weight: _____

Start Date: _____   Height: _____

	Initial Test	Retest 1	Retest 2	Retest 3
Right Arm (7 inches up from elbow)				
Left Arm				
Chest (across nipple line)				
Waist (across belly button)				
Hips (across bony prominences)				
Right Thigh (midpoint up from top of kneecap)				
Left Thigh				
Right Calf (up from ankle bone—largest section)				
Left Calf				

BODY FAT (TO BE MEASURED BY A SKILLED PROFESSIONAL)

Age: _____

	Initial Test	Retest 1	Retest 2	Retest 3
Chest* (men only)				
Abdomen (men only)				
Thigh (men and women)				
Hip (women only)				
Triceps (women only)				
Sum (mm)				
Percent Body Fat				

OTHER IMPORTANT MEASUREMENTS

Blood Pressure				
Resting Heart Rate (beats per minute at rest)				
Body Mass Index				
Waist to Hip Ratio				

*All measurements should be made in millimeters.

Body Measurements

It's important to measure just about every area of your body because if you tend to hold more fat in certain areas, like your upper arms, for instance, and have less around your thighs or waist, you'll be missing out on the joy of seeing your numbers drop.

Buy a tape measure that has a self-locking feature and will not stretch. This way you can take the measurements yourself with accuracy. Do not measure over clothing. Record the following measurements on your score sheet.

Arms. Measure 7 inches up from your bent elbow on your right arm—this should be about mid-bicep. Then wrap the tape around your arm at that 7-inch mark. Let it lock and hold. If it is 13 inches, for example, record 13 inches on the score sheet as your right arm measurement. Then measure your left arm the same way.

Chest. Wrap the tape around your chest across the nipple line. Take a deep breath in and let it out, then record the measurement in that neutral position.

Waist. Wrap the tape across your belly button line, being sure that the tape is at the same level in the back of your body as it is in the front. Do not pull the tape too hard. It should be snug but not too tight. Record that number.

Hips. With your feet touching each other, wrap the tape around the largest section of your hip area. This is usually across the two bony parts at the front of your body. Record the number.

Thigh. With your feet slightly more than hip-width apart, measure from the top of your kneecap to your mid-thigh. Record that number as the "site" of measurement. Then wrap the tape around your thigh until it is snug and record that number. Repeat on the other side.

Calves. Measure up from the top of the ankle bone on the outside of your leg to the largest part of your calf muscle. This is usually 9

Cut the Fat: The Facts about Body-Fat Testing

Body composition is really what the weight-loss game is all about. Here's a survey of the most common forms of body-fat testing, and what you need to know about each:

Skin-Fold Measurements

What is it? This is the most common form of body-fat testing. A handheld instrument called a caliper, generally the Lange type, measures the thickness of a pinch of skin on either three or seven sites on the body, such as the thigh, abdomen, triceps, and chest.

Accuracy: Done correctly, it is very accurate; the more sites, the better.

Cost: Often free.

Where to get tested: By personal trainers or at a health club, a school, a YMCA, a fitness center, a hospital, or a health fair.

Underwater Weighing

What is it? Sometimes called *hydrostatic weighing*, this method uses a "dunk tank" to measure water displacement. First you are weighed outside the tank, then you are submerged in it and weighed again underwater. If you have more bone and muscle, you'll weigh more in water than a person with less bone and muscle. In other words, higher body density equals a lower percentage of body fat. Since fat floats, a large amount of it will make the body lighter in water and show a higher percentage of body fat.

Accuracy: It's very accurate when done correctly. Since air makes the body float, you must blow all the air out of the lungs when you are weighed—both in water and out—otherwise, reliability drops.

Cost: $10 to $75.

Where to get tested: Testing isn't widely available because few places have the proper facilities, but some research institutions, wellness centers, and colleges offer it.

Bioelectrical Impedance Analysis (BIA)

What is it? BIA uses a very small electrical signal to measure fat, lean mass, and water. In general, fat causes the most "impedance," or resistance, to the signal because it contains less water than muscle. In conventional BIA, you lie down, and electrodes and conductive jelly are placed on a wrist and an ankle. A newer form of BIA, the Tanita method, is more convenient and easier to find. With Tanita, you stand on what looks like a bathroom scale and the current passes through your feet. In either case, the current is low and doesn't hurt.

Accuracy: This method can be fairly reliable, but only when done correctly. You must abstain from eating and drinking for at least 4 hours before testing and avoid exercise and also alcohol. Dehydration will seriously skew the results on this test, making it unreliable.

Cost: Free or up to $30.

Where to get tested: Fitness centers, health clubs, universities, health fairs, and doctor's and chiropractor's offices.

BOD POD

What is it? This is what it sounds like: a body pod. While you sit in an egglike chamber, a machine measures the volume of air the body displaces. With this data, body fat and lean mass can be calculated. The pod has a large acrylic window to prevent claustrophobia.

Accuracy: The company says that the range of error is very low—1 to 2 percent, similar to underwater measurements.

Cost: $30 to $100.

Where to get tested: You can get measured at hospitals, universities, and fitness centers, but in general, this testing isn't easy to come by.

or 10 inches from the top of the ankle bone. Record that number as the site of measurement. Then wrap the tape around the calf and record that number on your score sheet. Repeat with the other leg.

Body Fat

Body-fat testing is my favorite way to track progress because unlike the scale, it really shows if you're successful in turning your once sluggish metabolism into a fat-burning furnace. Building muscle increases your metabolism; in fact, you can burn an additional 50 calories a day just by adding one pound of muscle to your body. If you know what your body fat is from the start, you'll easily be able to measure your success.

In a nutshell, here's how to understand body fat:

	Women	Men
Athlete	10 to 15%	6 to 10%
Normal	15 to 25%	10 to 20%
Overweight	25.1 to 29.9%	20.1 to 24.9%
Obese	Over 30%	Over 25%

It's important to find a skilled trainer who can accurately measure your body fat. Testing body fat is tricky, and you want to be sure you use the same technician and the same method each time.

The most common method uses skin-fold calipers (the Lange model is the most popular) and measures fat beneath the outer layer of skin. There are many other forms of testing body fat, but some are costly or hard to find. It's important to record each skin-fold number (in millimeters) that corresponds to the site being measured and then the total sum (in millimeters) in the body-fat section of your score sheet. The person doing this test will be able to tell you what your overall body fat is. Record that number.

Other Measurements

The next three measurements are best done on calculators. You can find them all over the Web. It's easiest to visit the tools and calculators area on my Web site, www.ginalombardi.com.

Body Mass Index (BMI). Some people use Body Mass Index, or BMI, as a substitute for body-fat testing. But honestly, it's not an accurate measure of body fat, especially if you're in good shape. It can, however, give you a number that will tell you if you fall in or out of the range for good health. So I ask you to both measure body fat and calculate your BMI on my Web site by entering your height and weight.

BMI ranges look like this:

Less than 18.5%: Underweight

18.5 to 24.9%: Normal

25.0 to 29.9%: Overweight

Over 30%: Obese

Over 40%: Morbidly obese

Waist-to-Hip Ratio (WHR). This measurement compares the size of your waist to that of your hips and tells you how much fat is distributed around your midsection. Once you take the measurements, you can also calculate this number at my Web site, www.ginalombardi.com. To measure, wrap a nonstretchy measuring tape around your waist, making sure that it is level and parallel to the floor. Tighten it without squeezing the skin. Be sure to measure your waist at its narrowest point width-wise, usually just above the belly button. Then measure your hips around the widest part over the hip bones. Go to the online calculator, then record your number on the score sheet.

Important Note: Remember that BMI and WHR should be used only if you are more than 10 pounds overweight. If you consider yourself pretty fit, these methods of assessment will not be very accurate. So if you need to lose 10 pounds or less, leave this area blank.

Training Heart Rate. Your training heart rate tells you how vigorously you need to exercise in order to burn fat and improve cardiovascular fitness. It compares your resting heart rate—the number of times your heart beats per minute when you're relaxed—with how hard your heart is beating during exercise. This number also helps you monitor your fitness. As you get in shape, your resting heart rate will lower, so your training heart rate will change accordingly. To measure it most accurately, you would need an exercise physiologist or a physician to administer a VO2 max test, but that's not necessary for our purposes.

To figure out your training heart rate, you'll need your pulse rate. Feel for your pulse on your wrist, right below the base of the thumb, or on the side of your neck on the carotid artery (do not press too hard!). Count the beats for a full minute. *Do not* count for 10 seconds and multiply. Ideally, your true resting heart rate should be measured when you are sleeping and unable to actually take it, but you can get pretty close by taking your pulse in the morning before you get out of bed. An average resting heart rate is 50 to 80 beats per minute, and it rises with age.

Now that you know your resting heart rate, use my online calculator to find your training heart rate. Depending on your current fitness level, you'll want to work out at between 55 and 85 to 90 percent of your max. We will use these numbers later in this book to make up your training "range," depending on which program you are on.

You've figured out how much weight you'd like to lose and how much time you have, and you've got *all* your statistics recorded, so you're ready to go. It may have been a little time-consuming, but you will be thankful later when you can see your measurable results.

5

> > > >

Preparing for the Deadline

Don't be satisfied accepting where you are when where you could be is beautiful.

—Judy Mae

By now you probably have figured out that in order to succeed and meet your deadline, you need to change both your eating habits and your exercise habits. To me, it's not even fifty-fifty . . . each one is worth 100 percent in the "looking good" equation. And now that you have used the previous chapters to choose your realistic goal, learn why you're in the condition you're in, gather and record all your stats (otherwise known as measurements), you're *more* than ready to start the challenge and meet whichever deadline you select. And by the way, I know you can do it.

In a minute, you're going to turn to the chapter that corresponds to your own deadline. But in the meantime, no matter how much time you have, here is a checklist that includes everything you need to do to get started:

1. Make sure you've taken and recorded all of your measurements correctly. Keep your paperwork in a safe place, since you'll soon be using it to evaluate your progress.

2. Post your goals in a central spot so you can remind yourself why you wanted to lose weight in the first place.

3. Calculate the number of calories you can have each day in order to lose weight. It's a little involved, but you must have this number before you can put together a food plan. Step-by-step, here's how to do it:

   • Calculate your basal metabolic rate, or BMR, which is how many calories you need per day to maintain your current weight, using the online calculator in the tools and calculators section of my Web site, www.ginalombardi.com.

   • Figure out your total caloric requirement (TCR) by factoring in exercise. Your BMR multiplied by your activity level equals your TCR.

Lightly Active	You engage in everyday normal activity only	1.3
Moderately Active	You exercise three to four times a week for at least 30 minutes each session	1.4
Very Active	You exercise more than four times a week for 30 or more minutes each session	1.6
Extremely Active	You exercise six to seven times a week for 60 minutes or more each session	1.8

So if your BMR is 1,490 and you're moderately active, multiply 1,490 by 1.4. To maintain your weight when exercising, you'll need 2,086 calories per day.

   • Calculate your adjusted total calories to tell you what you can eat in order to lose weight. Subtract 500 calories from your total caloric requirement (2,086 minus 500 equals 1,586). This is how many calories you can consume in order to lose weight and fat. No matter what, don't consume fewer than 1,200 calories per day!

4. Be sure you've purchased everything you need in order to make this process easy for yourself (see the shopping lists on pages 59–61). Stock your fridge and cabinets with foods from the list I have provided in the chapter that corresponds with your chosen deadline.

5. Decide where you're going to work out and then do the following:

- If you plan to work out at the gym, get current with your membership.

- If you prefer a home-based workout with some equipment, buy the minimal amount. As you'll find in the coming chapters, I have all kinds of workouts for you—at the gym, using home equipment, and using *no* equipment at all. So there's no excuse. There is *always* a way for you to get a great workout.

>>> Talar's Story

Ever since I got married three and a half years ago, I've been putting on the extra pounds. Before the wedding, I lived at home, and my mother did all the cooking. Because I never really cooked, my husband and I ended up eating out a lot or getting takeout. We both work long hours and get home late—but we love to eat. So we basically lived on Chinese or whatever was easiest and a lot of junk food.

Luckily, I've always been good about exercise. I had a trainer and would work out twice a week. But it wasn't enough. Between the food and lack of the right exercise plan, I gained almost 40 pounds.

In the past, when I wanted to lose weight, I'd just stop eating. Gina taught me something different. Instead of always winging it—and then going on a drastic diet—I learned to make food a priority. That meant planning meals, rather than letting myself get hungry and then going for the first thing. I needed to get organized, go shopping, and be prepared for mealtime.

My program is very structured, three meals and two snacks, which is good for me. Though I never used to eat in the morning, I now get up early and make breakfast, usually choosing from a list of suggestions Gina gave me. I prefer egg whites, fat-free cheese, and a wheat tortilla. Or a protein shake and some cucumber slices.

For dinner, I have something like grilled chicken with steamed vegetables and maybe some brown rice or wheat pasta and a little olive oil.

I also added more exercise. I work out four times a week, with light weights and cardio for 45 minutes. I prefer the StairMaster, biking, or the elliptical trainer.

> **❝** So far, so good. I've lost 12 pounds, and my clothes have started to fit. **❞**
> —TALAR

Tips for Success

Yes, you can lose weight and get in shape on my programs. Here's how to ensure success:

- Stick to the program exactly. It took me fifteen years to perfect these plans, and they work . . . if you follow them precisely. Adding items to the list, skipping meals, adding meals, or eating out a lot will *not* give you good results. Now is the time to buckle down and do it.

- Post your goals sheet in a central spot so that you can constantly remind yourself why you decided to get on the program in the first place. Then take it seriously!

- Get your family ready. Make sure they support and encourage you. This is another key to your success. Include your children in your workouts or arrange for child care if you have to.

- Start off on the right foot with a good pair of comfortable, supportive shoes and well-

made, breathable workout clothing. See the sidebars on page 61 for tips on how to choose a good shoe and advice on buying the right workout clothing.

- Always warm up by starting your exercise session with 5 to 10 minutes of any type of aerobic exercise, such as walking, jogging, cycling—even jumping jacks. You don't need to stretch before weight training. (If you'd like to stretch, do it at the end of your session.) It's better to do a "warm-up set." Simply perform the exercise for one set with a very light load, about half of the weight you would typically use. This will improve blood flow to the muscles you will be exercising.

- Always cool down. A cool-down period will help the body remove the by-products (such as lactic acid) that accumulate in the muscle

So far so good. I've lost 12 pounds and my clothes have started to fit. I'm beginning to get comments from my family and friends, and my husband thinks I look great. <<<

Eating Plan Shopping List

Before you get going, you'll need:

- A digital kitchen food scale
- A digital bathroom scale (not the kind that measures body fat—they are not accurate)
- A blender and/or a sturdy shaker cup
- A 32-ounce refillable water bottle
- A heart-rate monitor
- Protein powders and supplements

tissue during training by moving them back into the bloodstream, where they are processed and removed by the body. Simply spend 5 to 10 minutes walking, cycling, or performing any other type of aerobic exercise (as in the warm-up) to help clear these waste products.

- Schedule time for your workouts and for preparing meals. Be sure that you arrange your schedule to fit your new healthy lifestyle, whether it's getting up earlier to work out or going to your job later in the morning, working out at lunch with a buddy or hitting the gym on your way home. Carve out the time and commit to it!

- At times when you feel the urge to go off the eating plan, remember your goal. Look at it. Recommit to sticking to this plan. This is a true test of discipline. The one thing that no one can ever take away from you is your ability to control your thoughts and your actions. Make good choices!

- If you feel you are not getting the results you should, run through the "debug" checklist in each deadline chapter. If something isn't working, that means you're doing something that's not on the program. Find it and fix it.

- Every four to six weeks, retest your body fat and measurements as directed and record them on your score sheet. Take your measurements the exact same way you did for the initial testing. If you had someone test your body fat, go back to that same person and have him or her do the retest. This will ensure accuracy.

Exercise Plan Shopping List

Here's what you'll need for workouts at home:

Dumbbells. These should vary in weight increments. Depending on your current level of strength, choose pairs of 5 pounds up to pairs of 30 pounds for most women and up to 50 pounds or more for some men.

Stability Ball. See the sizing chart below to choose the right size ball for you.

If Your Height Is:	You Need This Ball
Up to four feet ten	Small (45 centimeters = 18 inches)
Four feet ten to five feet five	Medium (55 centimeters = 22 inches)
Five feet five to six feet	Large (65 centimeters = 26 inches)
Six feet to six feet five	X-large (75 centimeters = 30 inches)
Over six feet five	XX-Large (85 centimeters = 33 inches)

Note: This chart offers a general guide. It's best to choose a ball that allows you to sit with your knees and hips at 90 degrees (thighs parallel to the floor). Using different-size balls to accommodate individual needs or to vary the difficulty of the exercises is okay, too. In fact, the smaller the ball, the more difficult the exercise.

Plyometric Boxes.* These come 12 inches high and 18 inches high. They are generally for advanced exercisers.

36-inch Foam Roll. For intermediate and advanced exercisers.

Medicine Ball. The weight will depend on your current fitness level. Start with a 10-pound ball and move up from there.

Weighted Bar (optional) These bars come in varying weights from 3 pounds up to 20 pounds and can be used in place of dumbbells or barbells for variety.

Cushioned Mat. To protect your spine if you are lying down, especially if you are on a hardwood floor.

Shoes. Select a good pair of cross-training, walking, and/or running shoes (see the sidebar on page 61).

Clothing. Breathable, moisture-wicking workout clothing is best (see the sidebar on page 61).

*Go to www.power-systems.com to purchase the equipment on this page.

A Shoe-in

If it's time for a new pair of athletic shoes, follow these tips:

- Choose shoes that fit the activity or activities you will be participating in: walking shoes for walking; running shoes for running, cross-trainers for weight lifting and classes, hiking shoes for hiking. Get the idea? Each shoe is specifically engineered for those activities. Each should have proper and appropriate flexibility, good arch support, and a heel that's right for the sport or activity. For instance, choose a low heel for walking to prevent lower-back pain.
- Regarding the toe box, be sure there's a half inch of room between the end of your big toe and the tip of the shoe.
- To get the right fit, go to a boutique store that will provide personalized attention. If you're shopping for running shoes, for example, visit a store that specializes in running equipment.

The salesperson should measure your foot and take you outside to evaluate you as you walk or run in order to suggest a shoe that fits your individual needs.

- Choose a sock that is padded in the heel, arch, and ball of the foot for added cushioning and comfort. It should be a blend of acrylic, nylon, and spandex but not cotton alone. This will help prevent blistering and keep your feet drier.
- Shoes can range from $40 at discount stores to $150 at full retail. Shoes in the $80 to $90 price range are usually your best bet for a quality, longer-lasting product.
- If you have wide or extra-wide feet, go with a brand that has E and EE widths.
- Once you purchase your new shoes, use a permanent marker to write the date on the inside of the shoe tongue. After six months or 500 miles, whichever comes first, it's time for a new pair of shoes!

The Clothes Call

Quality workout clothing is a must. Here are some tips:

For Men and Women

- Choose a moisture-wicking fabric like Coolmax or Thinsulate to keep skin dry.
- In cold weather, layer clothing first with a light T-shirt followed by a light long-sleeved shirt or long underwear, then a sweatshirt. For rainy weather, invest in waterproof shoes and a water-resistant jacket.
- For serious fitness enthusiasts, try Skins to reduce soreness, recovery time, and fatigue. Go to www.skins.net.

Women Only

- Motion can cause traditional bra hooks to unhook, so select a sports bra that has a racer back or T-back type of strap design. These will not only give you better support but will also prevent the straps from slipping off your shoulders. Wider straps can help distribute weight, resulting in less digging in. Make sure the bra is made of a wicking fabric like Coolmax, polypropylene, or Thinsulate. Wet cotton is virtually impossible to get off after a workout. Notice whether fabric becomes see-through when wet. This is an embarrassment none of us needs. You can even choose a style that doubles as a nice top and can be worn outside the gym as well.
- My favorite hairbands and headbands are by i/m Studio. They are fashionable and really hold your hair together, even with vigorous exercise like boxing, kickboxing, and dance classes!

Enhancing Your Deadline Program

Taking certain supplements may help you lose weight faster. But you may be confused about whether to take them or which ones work best.

Overall, taking supplements is a smart idea, especially on a weight-loss program. Vitamins and minerals help ensure that you get all of the nutrients you need and also play a supporting role in the metabolic processes of the body. There are three levels of supplementation for you to consider: basics, extras, and weight loss.

It's great for everyone to take a vitamin and mineral supplement that provides everything on my basics list. For even more of a health boost, see my extras list. If you can find a supplement that has it all— great. If not, simply add the extras to your daily vitamin/mineral supplement.

You can enhance your deadline results by adding one or more of the weight-loss supplements to your program. Once you have reached your goal, drop the weight-loss supplements, except for green tea; you can keep that one for life.

With all supplements, including green tea, check with your doctor before taking them, particularly if you're on any medications that they might interact with. Here's a list of common supplements and their dosages.

The Basics (Daily Doses)

Vitamin A	5,000 to 10,000 international units
Beta-carotene (natural form)	5,000 to 10,000 international units
B complex	25 to 100 milligrams
Boron	1 to 3 milligrams
Calcium	500 to 1000 milligrams
Chromium	50 to 200 micrograms
Copper	2 milligrams

Vitamin D	400 to 1000 international units
Vitamin E (D-alpha)	400 to 800 international units
Iodine	150 micrograms
Iron (optional)	8 to 18 milligrams
Magnesium	250 to 500 milligrams
Manganese	5 to 15 milligrams
Selenium	50 to 200 micrograms
Zinc	15 to 25 milligrams

Check with your physician or nutritionist to decide if iron supplementation is important for you, especially if you are pregnant. The recommended daily intake is currently 8 milligrams a day for males, 18 milligrams a day for females, and 27 milligrams a day for pregnant women, 8 milligrams a day for men and women over 51 years of age.

As a general rule, take supplements with food to enhance absorption and guard against upset stomach. If your multivitamin/mineral requires more than one pill per day, take half with one meal and half with another meal. Be sure to store all your supplements in a cool (or at least room-temperature), dark place. Sunlight can decrease the effectiveness of some ingredients. Don't refrigerate supplements unless the bottle tells you to do so. Yes, the environment is cool, but it is also damp . . . another problem. If you carry supplements to work or while traveling, keep them in their original containers or in a dark, airtight bottle.

Extras

Fish Oil. Hands down, fish oil is probably the most important extra you could take. Omega-3 fatty acids, specifically EPA (eicosapentanoic acid) and DHA (docosahexanoic acid), help heat the body, lower triglycerides, decrease clotting, lower blood pressure, reduce inflammation, and even stabilize mood. They are so beneficial that the FDA recently allowed manufacturers to print health claims for them on labels.

CoEnzyme Q-10. This powerful antioxidant has loads of benefits, including the prevention and/or treatment of cardiovascular disease, cancer, and immune problems. Although our bodies do produce some, we also lose it when we exercise. Taking 50 to 100 milligrams daily is good insurance that your body will continue to reap the benefits of this compound.

Chromium. As I mentioned earlier, insulin resistance is a growing problem that causes some people to have trouble controlling their weight. Chromium can help.

Studies show that at least 200 micrograms daily is needed to improve insulin resistance, but as much as 400 to 600 a day may be necessary for some people. (If you have type 2 diabetes and are on diabetes medication, check with your doctor before taking chromium. Your medication may have to be adjusted.)

Magnesium. This mineral is an often overlooked ingredient in the insulin-resistance mix. Although you may have some in your daily vitamin/mineral supplement, it may be beneficial to take in as much as 400 milligrams a day to help you with any carbohydrate sensitivity you may have.

The Truth about Caffeine

Caffeine is often recommended as a weight-loss supplement. Here are the pros and cons:

Pros

- It stimulates the central nervous system, thereby revving up metabolism and increasing mental alertness.
- It can increase metabolic rate by approximately 10 percent with as little as 100 to 150 milligrams (the amount in a typical cup of coffee) periodically throughout the day (because of these properties it is often coupled with other weight-loss supplements to achieve even greater results).

- When combined with some ingredients, caffeine can lose some of its stimulating effects and become more tolerable.

Cons

- Because it is a stimulant, caffeine increases heart rate, causing jitters. It can cause breast sensitivity and digestive upset in some people and might lead to leaching of important minerals like calcium.
- If you have high blood pressure, a heart condition, insomnia, or caffeine intolerance, it is best to steer clear of caffeine entirely.

Weight-Loss Supplements

You probably know from magazine and radio ads that there are now many supplements that claim to enhance weight loss. However, no supplement melts off fat without you doing any work. There are supplements that can assist your body with metabolic issues that may be keeping you from losing weight. Here are some that have stood the test of time and research:

Important Reminder: Tell your doctor about any supplements you wish to take. Some supplements may interact with a medication you are taking or a condition you may have.

What is it	Function	Daily Dose
Chitosan	Fat blocker	500 to 1500 milligrams a day, at the start of a meal
Citrus aurantium	Metabolic booster	500 to 975 milligrams a day plus 500 milligrams caffeine
Coleus Forskohlii	Metabolic booster	25 milligrams twice a day before meals
Green tea	Metabolic booster	90 milligrams standardized EGCG three times a day
GSE	Carb regulator	400 milligrams
HCA	Metabolic booster	1000 to 3000 milligrams
L-Carnitine	Metabolic booster	500 to 2000 milligrams before your workout
Pyruvate	Metabolic booster	3 grams twice a day taken before meals
Redline*	Metabolic booster and mood enhancer	4 ounces liquid a day

*Go to www.upxsports.com for more information before using this product.

Now you're ready to roll. Turn to the chapter with *your* deadline instructions.

6

>>>>

Three Months and Counting

Above all, try something.

—*Franklin D. Roosevelt*

Three months is a gift! Lots of people come to me with only a couple of weeks to make changes in their bodies. Your main focus during these ninety days should be to make specific but gradual adjustments in the way you eat and exercise so that the change doesn't feel overwhelming. I hate the word *deprived*, and you shouldn't feel that way on this deadline. With more time, you'll be able to enjoy a lot of things you love, as long as you eat them in smaller amounts and avoid overindulging. By making good food choices and sticking to a workable exercise plan, you will get the body you want right on time.

But it's up to you. I've worked with hundreds of clients, and results always vary from person to person. A few exceeded the best possible results, and one or two fell slightly below the low end of possible results. How can this be? The answer is simple. Results equal the effort, time, and discipline you are willing to commit to. Period.

>>> Kristie's Story

Ever since I was about fourteen, I've had issues with portions and self-control. I'm an emotional eater, so I tend to eat when I'm bored or sad or whatever. Plus, I have never been into sports or working out. I'd rather sit down, play a video game, and eat a cheeseburger than work out and have a salad.

Near the end of last January, though, I reached a breaking point. I'm about five foot nine, and I had gotten up to 174 pounds. Some of my college classmates and I were planning a summer trip to Spain to study Spanish for a month, so I decided I wanted to lose weight for that trip. That's when I started working with Gina.

> 66 I used to think it was okay to diet for a while and then go back to my old habits. But what I learned is that dieting isn't short term. Eating healthy is supposed to stick with you forever. 99
> —KRISTIE

Right off, I had to change the way I ate. Normally, I'd skip breakfast, which was really bad. To get my metabolism more regulated, I started eating four meals a day, spaced out by about 3 to 4 hours. I chose what to eat from a list of foods, broken down by protein, veggies, fat, and carbs, and I had to portion out and weigh everything.

I was surprised at how easy that ended up being. I never felt like I was depriving myself, because I got to eat so often. And there were so many foods on the list that I could always make something good out of what was available to me. I would cheat, but only rarely.

The exercise wasn't so bad either. Though I had always been sedentary, working out felt good. At the beginning, I stuck to just cardio, mainly walking on the treadmill, sometimes with steep inclines and intervals. After the first month, I had lost 14 pounds, which was really motivating. I knew that if I kept doing it, I would lose more and more and more. Eventually I progressed to jogging, added weight training, and also signed up at a gym for martial arts classes. It wasn't too long before I was exercising six days a week.

By the three-month mark, I had lost almost 30 pounds, and just before I left for Spain, I was down to 141. On this program, I learned some good habits. I used to think it was okay to diet for a while and then go back to my old habits. But what I learned is that dieting isn't short term. Eating healthy is supposed to stick with you forever. <<<

<table>
<tr><td>the
EATING
Game Plan
at a
Glance</td><td>

Step 1 Pull out the adjusted total calories, or ATC, that you calculated in chapter 5. This tells you how much you can eat and still lose weight.

Step 2 Choose an eating plan, A or B, depending on how many times a day you prefer to eat.

Step 3 Using one of the caloric worksheets on pages 70–75, outline the makeup of your meals—how many calories you will consume in each meal and the protein, fat, nonstarchy vegetables, and complex carbohydrate breakdowns of each.

Step 4 Pull it all together: look over the food lists and plug in protein, fat, nonstarchy vegetable, and complex carb choices.

</td></tr>
</table>

Your Custom Eating Plan

First you need to decide which plan works best in your busy schedule. Here are your choices:

Plan A: Four meals a day

Plan B: Three meals a day plus two minisnacks

It doesn't matter which plan you choose because the calories are the same. But if it's easier, for example, for you to plan three meals and sneak in two minisnacks, go with that plan instead of the four-meal plan. Either way, the goal is to feed the machine constantly to keep your metabolism at optimum speed. Skipping meals or snacks will not get you there faster, so don't even think about it.

Plan A: Four Meals a Day

You should know your adjusted total calories (ATC)—how many calories you can consume and still lose weight—from chapter 5. So let's calculate how many calories should make up each meal. We will further break down the calories in each meal by protein, fat, non-starchy veggies, and complex carbs. Remember, grams of carbs refers to a combination of veggies and complex carbs.

Plan A Caloric Worksheet

_____ ATC ÷ 4 meals = _____ calories/meal

CARBS

_____ calories/meal × 45% = _____ carbohydrate calories/meal

_____ carbohydrate calories/meal ÷ 4* = _____ carbohydrate grams/meal

*There are 4 calories per gram of carbs.

PROTEIN

_____ calories/meal × 35% = _____ protein calories/meal

_____ protein calories/meal ÷ 4* = _____ protein grams/meal

*There are 4 calories per gram of protein.

FAT

_____ calories/meal × 20% = _____ fat calories/meal

_____ fat calories/meal ÷ 9* = _____ fat grams/meal

*There are 9 calories per gram of fat.

Grams of carbs   = _____ /meal
Grams of protein = _____ /meal
Grams of fat   = _____ /meal

To build your meals, use the list below to combine (per meal):

One lean protein item

One healthy fat item

One nonstarchy vegetable item

One complex carb item

Lean Proteins

Choose one for each meal.

- Egg white, scrambled or hard-boiled (1 large egg white = 4 grams; 1 cup = 26 grams)

- Fish—always your best choice; see my best and worst fish guide in chapter 2 (1 ounce = 6 grams)

- Lean beef, 7 percent fat—limit to two to three times a week) (1 ounce = 9 grams)

- Nonfat cheese—mozzarella, string, etc. (1 ounce = 9 grams)

- Nonfat cottage cheese (1 ounce = 5 grams; 1 cup = 25 grams)

- 100 percent pure microfiltered ion-exchanged whey protein isolate powders, with less than 5 grams carbs and no fat (1 scoop = 20 grams)

- Other meats: turkey bacon (1 ounce cooked = 5 grams); fat-free/nitrate-free chicken or turkey sausage (1 ounce = 4 grams), venison (1 ounce = 7 grams), buffalo (1 ounce = 8 grams)

- Skinless, boneless chicken or turkey breast (1 ounce = 6 grams)

- Soy hot dogs and burgers, fat-free type (1 ounce = 6 grams)

- Tofu—silken, light, or extra firm (1 ounce = 2 grams)

Healthy Fats

Choose one for each meal.

- Avocado (1 ounce = 4 grams)

- Black or green olives (1 ounce = 4 grams)

- Cream cheese, whipped (1 tablespoon = 3 grams)

- Dark chocolate, low carb—limit to three times a week (1 ounce = 9 grams)

- Hummus (1 tablespoon = 1 gram)

- Nuts—about nine almonds, cashews, walnuts, or peanuts (½ ounce = 8 grams)

- Olive oil, flax oil, safflower oil, tahini, sunflower oil (1 teaspoon = 5 grams)
- Organic butter (1 tablespoon = 11 grams)
- Peanut butter or almond butter (1 tablespoon = 8 grams)
- Regular salad dressing (1 tablespoon = 8 grams)
- Soy, safflower, or canola mayonnaise, light versions (1 tablespoon = 5 grams)

Nonstarchy Lower-Carb Vegetables

Choose one for each meal, steamed. Or you can mix two or three together if you prefer.

- Artichoke hearts (½ cup = 13 grams)
- Asparagus (1 spear = 1 gram)
- Bamboo Shoots (1 cup = 2 grams)
- Broccoli (1 cup = 6 grams)
- Brussels sprouts (1 cup = 8 grams)
- Cabbage (1 cup = 5 grams)
- Cauliflower (1 cup cooked = 5 grams)
- Celery and celery root (1 cup = 3 grams)
- Cucumbers or pickles with no added sugars (1 cup = 3 grams)
- Eggplant (1 cup cooked = 8 grams)
- Fennel (1 cup = 6 grams)
- Green beans, wax beans, and sprouts (1 cup = 8 grams)
- Greens—lettuces, spinach, chard, etc. (1 cup = 2 grams)
- Hearty greens, such as kale, collards, mustard greens, etc. (1 cup = 8 grams)
- Herbs—basil, cilantro, parsley, rosemary, thyme, etc.
- Jicama (1 cup = 11 grams)
- Leeks (1 cup = 13 grams)
- Mushrooms (1 cup = 2 grams)
- Okra (1 cup = 7 grams)
- Onions (1 cup = 15 grams)
- Peppers, all colors and kinds (12 grams per whole large pepper)
- Radicchio and endive (1 cup = 8 grams)
- Radishes (1 cup = 4 grams)
- Sea vegetables—nori, seaweed, etc. (⅛ cup = 1 gram)

- Scallions or green onions (½ cup = 3 grams)
- Snow peas (1 cup = 7 grams)
- Summer Squash (1 cup = 4 grams)
- Tomatoes (1 medium = 5 grams)
- Turnip (1 cup = 8 grams)
- Water chestnuts (1 cup = 17 grams)
- Zucchini (1 cup = 4 grams)

Complex Carbs
Choose one for each meal

- Apple (1 cup slices = 25 grams), peach (1 cup slices = 15 grams), pear (1 cup slices = 22 grams), plum (1 cup slices = 19 grams), grapefruit (1 cup slices = 19 grams), orange (1 cup slices = 21 grams), nectarine (1 cup slices = 15 grams), cantaloupe or honeydew (1 cup balls = 16 grams), strawberries, blueberries, raspberries, blackberries (1 cup = 12 grams)
- Cooked brown rice (1 cup = 45 grams)
- High-fiber cereal, such as Fiber One, with ½ cup nonfat organic milk (½ cup cereal = 25 grams; ½ cup nonfat milk = 7 grams)
- Lavash (1½ ounce = 23 grams)
- Quick oats (dry) (½ cup = 27 grams)
- Whole grain bread (1 slice = 11 grams)
- Whole grain crackers—no trans fats (1 thin cracker = 1 gram)
- Whole grain pita or whole grain tortilla (4-inch size = 15 grams)
- Yam or sweet potato (1 cup = 37 grams)

*Nutritional data in parentheses was taken from www.nutritiondata.com.

Plan B: Three Meals with Two Snacks

For this plan, use your adjusted total calories (from chapter 5), then follow this worksheet to figure out how many calories—broken down by protein, fat, and the two kinds of carbohydrates (nonstarchy veggies and complex carbs)—should be in each meal and snack. Do not save both snacks for late-night grazing!

Plan B Caloric Worksheet

_____ ATC × 75% = _____ ÷ 3 meals/day = _____ calories/meal

CARBS PER MEAL

_____ calories/meal × 45% = _____ carbohydrate calories/meal

_____ carbohydrate calories/meal ÷ 4* = _____ carbohydrate grams/meal

There are 4 calories per gram of carbs.

PROTEIN PER MEAL

_____ calories/meal × 35% = _____ protein calories/meal

_____ protein calories/meal ÷ 4* = _____ protein grams/meal

There are 4 calories per gram of protein.

FAT PER MEAL

_____ calories/meal × 20% = _____ fat calories/meal

_____ fat calories/meal ÷ 9* = _____ fat grams/meal

There are 9 calories per gram of fat.

SNACKS

_____ ATC × 25% = _____ ÷ 2 snacks/day = _____ calories/snack

Carbs

_____ calories/snack × 55% = _____ carbohydrate calories/snack

_____ carbohydrate calories/meal ÷ 4* =_____ carbohydrate grams/snack

There are 4 calories per gram of carbs.

Protein

_____ calories/snack × 45% = _____ protein calories/snack

_____ protein calories/snack ÷ 4* =_____ protein grams/snack

There are 4 calories per gram of protein.

Meals		Snacks	
Grams of carbs = _____ /meal		Grams of carbs = _____ /snack	
Grams of protein = _____ /meal		Grams of protein = _____ /snack	
Grams of fat = _____ /meal			

Snack Attack

Good news: here are some healthy snacks you can munch on! Each consists of a protein and a carbohydrate. Remember to stick to the serving sizes you calculated in your plan's caloric worksheet on pages 71–73.

- Almonds, walnuts, or cashews and nonfat cheese
- Baked chips with fresh salsa and light mozzarella string cheese sticks
- Chicken breast slices and veggie chips
- Fat-free turkey breast slices and a 100-calorie bag of cheese crackers
- Fresh turkey slices or skinless chicken breast slices and 1 small apple
- Nonfat mozzarella cheese and berries
- Protein shake made with whey protein powder, ice, and water, plus berries
- Whey protein powder protein shake and crackers

Sweet Surprise

If you're desperate for sweets, enjoy ½ ounce dark chocolate (about five Special Dark Hershey's Kisses) with some light string cheese. But try not to indulge more than three times a week!

---

the **EXERCISE** Game Plan at a Glance	

Step 1 Determine your exercise level—beginner, intermediate, or advanced. Refer to chapter 3 ("What Kind of Shape Are You In?") to figure out your current fitness level.

Step 2 Look over the workout schedule. You'll do both cardio and resistance training several times a week. You can exercise with equipment or without. If you choose to use equipment, make sure you've got everything you need. I also offer suggestions on how to incorporate exercise machines for variety and convenience.

Step 3 Study the illustrations and descriptions of the resistance exercises. This will help you do the workouts properly.

Step 4 Put it all together: Be sure to do the proper progression by starting with weeks 1 through 4 at your appropriate exercise level. If you aren't ready to progress, it's also okay to stay on weeks 1 through 4 rather than progressing to weeks 5 through 8.

Important Note: Always check with your physician before starting a new exercise program, especially if you have any medical conditions.

Your Custom Exercise Program

Now that you've got your food formula, it's time to create your exercise plan. Using the guidelines in the box on page 75, choose the cardio and resistance exercise programs that best suit your current level of fitness.

Beginner Workouts

If you're a beginner, you will do this exercise program for twelve weeks, including the progressions. Once you can do those, you can move on to the intermediate programs.

Fit Tips for Beginners

You won't be a beginner for long. The beginner programs will give you a good base of strength and muscle stimulus necessary for the upcoming programs. Follow these suggestions for a better workout:

- Work out in the gym or at home with or without equipment, and stick to the plan. Move on only when it is comfortable for you or you feel you are not getting any more results from the workout you are doing.
- Take the time to look at the pictures and read the exercise descriptions to ensure proper technique.
- Always warm up for at least 5 minutes prior to weight training. For best results, stretch at the end of your session.
- Start with a weight that allows you to handle 8 to 12 repetitions with good form.
- Follow the weekly progressions (one set of each exercise the first four weeks, etc.).

- Take the rest periods of 1 to 2 minutes between sets and exercises.
- Perform each exercise in a smooth manner and through a full range of motion.
- Perform each exercise in the sequence it is written. Large muscle groups (such as the legs) are trained first because they require more energy, followed by smaller muscle groups (such as the arms).
- Don't be tempted to weight train on consecutive days. Keep a day in between for rest and recovery.
- Do cardio on alternating days as a general rule. If you have to do it on the same day as weight training, do it after your weight workout.
- The no equipment workouts can be very strenuous! Don't do them every day. Do your cardio on the alternating days instead.

Cardio

BEGINNER: WEEKS 1 THROUGH 8

- Warm up for 5 minutes.
- For weeks 1 through 4, do 20 minutes at 55 to 75 percent of HR max. For weeks 1 through 8, do 30 minutes at 55 to 75 percent HR max.
- Cool down for 5 minutes.
- Do cardio three times per week, alternating with days of weight training.

BEGINNER: WEEKS 9 THROUGH 12

- Warm up for 5 minutes at 55 to 75 percent HR max.
- Do 30 minutes: 15 minutes at 55 to 75 percent HR max, followed by 15 minutes of intervals as described on page 34.
- Do cardio three times per week, alternating with days of weight training.

Weight Training

BEGINNER: WEEKS 1 THROUGH 4

- Warm up with 5 to 10 minutes of continuous cardio exercise, such as walking or stair-climbing.
- Do one set of 8 to 12 repetitions per exercise.
- Allow 1 to 2 minutes of rest between sets.
- Train on three nonconsecutive days per week: Monday, Wednesday, Friday or Tuesday, Thursday, Saturday.

Dumbbell Squat

To start > Stand with a dumbbell in each hand. Look straight ahead, keeping your back straight, your arms straight at your sides, and your feet flat on the floor, with your weight equally distributed between your forefoot and your heel. Your knees should point in the same direction as your feet throughout the movement.

Action > Keeping your arms straight at your sides and slightly forward as shown, lower yourself until your thighs are parallel to the floor. Keep your back straight and look slightly upward to ensure that you don't slouch forward. Do not allow your knees to extend past your toes. Pause, then return to the starting position by pushing through the middle of your feet. Don't be tempted to go up on your toes or rock back on your heels, as you may lose your balance.

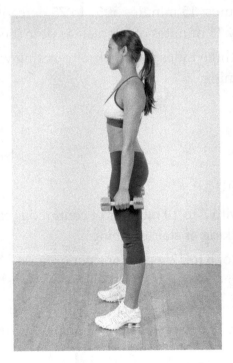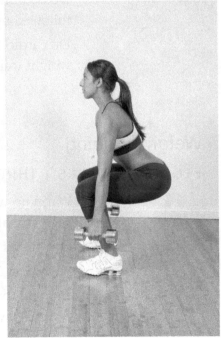

Stability Ball Leg Curl

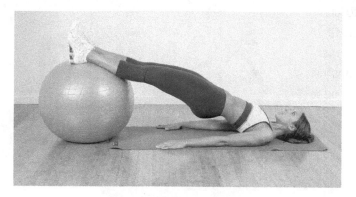

To start > Lie on your back on a cushioned floor or mat. Place the ball under your legs, between your knees and your feet. Raise your hips into the air as you push down into the ball. At the top of the lift, your body should be straight, at a 30-degree angle to the floor. Hold the position.

Action > Pull the ball in toward your glutes, keeping your hips off the floor. Bring it in as far as possible, then slowly release it back to the starting position.

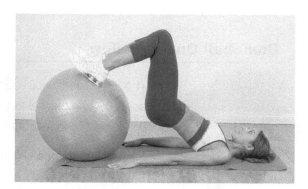

Dumbbell Bench Press

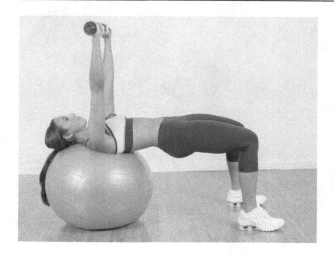

To start > Hold a dumbbell in each hand, keeping the weights close to your chest. Sit on the ball and roll down, walking your feet out in front of you until your head and upper back are resting on the ball. Straighten your arms out above your chest with your palms facing away from you. Keep your hips up and off the ball and your feet apart to maintain core stability.

Action › Lower the weights by bending at the elbow, being sure not to let the weights "buckle in" toward the center of your chest. Keep your forearms perpendicular to the floor. Lower your arms just below chest level, then press them up to the starting position.

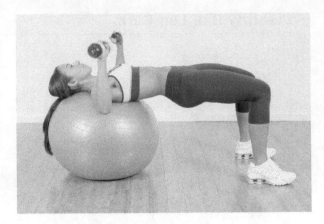

Dumbbell One-Arm Row

To start › Stand and place your left palm on a bench. Bend at the waist so that your back is flat and parallel to the floor. Your knees should be slightly bent and your neck should be in a neutral position.

Action › Holding a dumbbell in your right hand with your palm facing toward you, lift the dumbbell up to your rib cage area, elbow above waist. Return to the starting position.

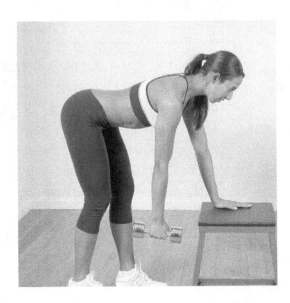
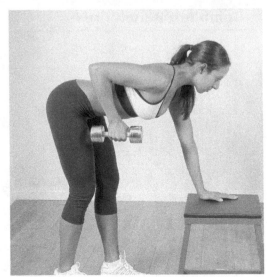

Dumbbell Biceps Curl

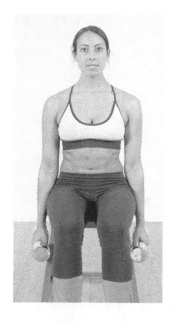 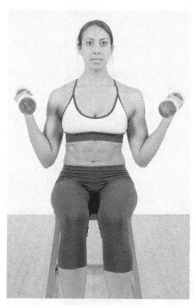

To start > Sit with a dumbbell in each hand, palms facing toward you and arms straight.

Action > Bend your elbows while rotating your forearms until they are vertical and your palms are facing your shoulders. Lower your arms to the starting position.

Dumbbell Triceps Kickback

To start > Holding a dumbbell in each hand, stand with a slight bend in your knees and bend at the waist about 45 degrees. Start with the dumbbells in front of you at chest level with your palms facing toward you. Look straight ahead and keep your neck in a neutral position.

Action > Extend your elbows until the dumbbells are behind you. Return to the starting position.

When you get this exercise down, you may try the Lying Dumbbell Triceps Extension variation on page 90.

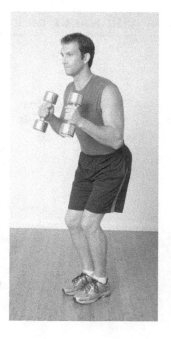 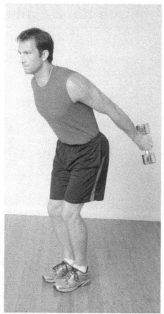

Abdominal Crunch

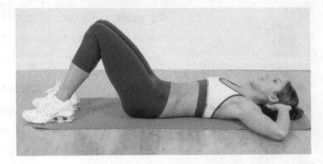

To start › Lie on your back on a mat with your knees bent and your feet flat on the floor. Lightly rest your fingertips on the back of your head.

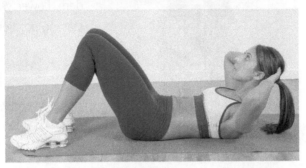

Action › Slowly curl your trunk forward, focusing on using your abdominal muscles, not your hands, to pull your head up.

Prone Back Extension with Hands on Lower Back

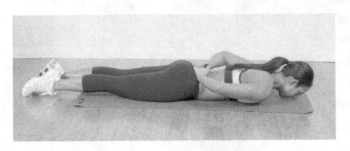

To start › Lie facedown on a mat with your hands on your lower back as shown.

Action › Raise your shoulders, chest, head, and legs smoothly as far up as you comfortably can. Keep your neck in line with your spine. Hold for 4 seconds, then slowly lower yourself back down.

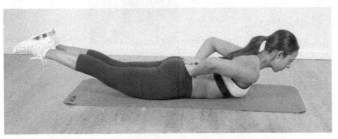

BEGINNER: WEEKS 5 THROUGH 8

- Warm up with 5 to 10 minutes of continuous cardio exercise, such walking or stair-climbing.
- Do two sets of 8 to 12 repetitions per exercise.
- Allow 1 to 2 minutes of rest between sets.
- Train on three nonconsecutive days per week: Monday, Wednesday, Friday or Tuesday, Thursday, Saturday.

Dumbbell Wall Squat with Stability Ball

To start > Place the ball against the wall and stand in front of it so that the ball is in contact with your lower middle back. Be sure to walk your feet out a little so that your knees will stay behind your toes when you go into the squat. You should be able to see your feet if you look down.

Action > Holding a dumbbell in each hand and keeping your arms at your sides, lower yourself until your thighs are parallel to the floor, or slightly lower if you can. Pause, then return to the starting position.

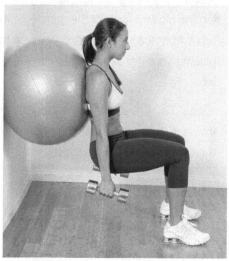

Gina's Tip: This is a perfect choice if you're a beginner, have back problems, or just want to vary your workout. The ball adds support for your back so you can squat a bit lower.

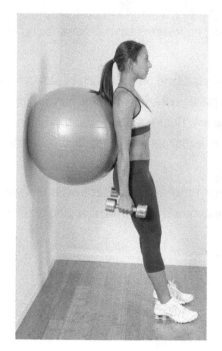

Dumbbell Step-Up on Bench or Step

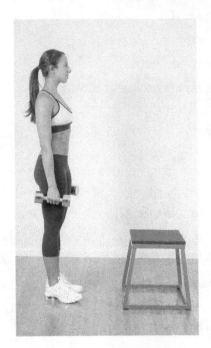 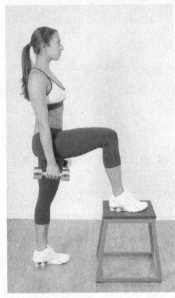 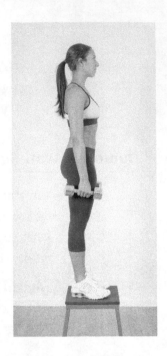

To start > Stand with a dumbbell in each hand, arms at your sides, facing the side of the bench.

Action > Place your right foot on the bench. Stand on the bench by straightening the hip and knee of the right leg and place your left foot on the bench slightly apart from the right. Step down with the left. Return to the starting position by placing your right foot on the floor. Do an equal number of repetitions on each leg.

Gina's Tip: Keep your torso upright during this exercise. Stepping a bit away from the bench works the butt (gluteus maximus) more, while stepping closer to the bench works the quadriceps.

> **Stability Ball Leg Curl** (page 79)

> **Dumbbell Bench Press** (page 79)

> **Dumbbell One-Arm Row** (page 80)

Dumbbell Lateral Raise

To start > Stand with a dumbbell in each hand, hands in front of your midsection. Slightly bend at the waist and keep your knees in a soft position.

Action > With your elbows slightly bent, raise your arms out to your sides until your elbows are shoulder height and slightly higher than your wrists, then lower yourself to the starting position.

Gina's Tip: Maintain a fixed elbow position (a 10- to 30-degree angle from your torso) throughout the exercise.

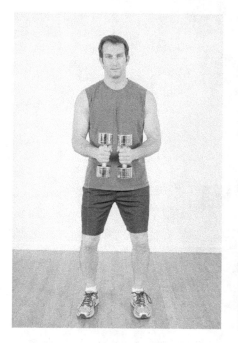 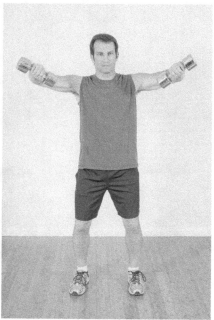

> **Dumbbell Biceps Curl** (page 81)

> **Dumbbell Triceps Kickback** (page 81)

> **Abdominal Crunch** (page 82)

One-Leg Hip Extension on All Fours, Alternating

To start ❯ Position yourself on all fours on a mat, keeping your neck in a neutral position as shown.

Action ❯ Extend one leg behind you, pause, then lower it to floor. Do an equal number of repetitions with each leg.

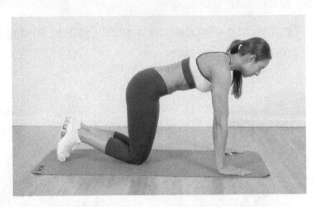

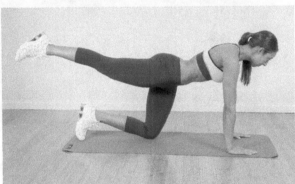

BEGINNER: WEEKS 9 THROUGH 12

- Warm up with 5 to 10 minutes of continuous cardio exercise, such as walking or stair-climbing.
- Do three sets of 8 to 12 repetitions per exercise.
- Allow 1 to 2 minutes of rest between sets.
- Train on three nonconsecutive days per week: Monday, Wednesday, Friday or Tuesday, Thursday, Saturday.

Dumbbell Walking Lunge

To start ❯ Stand with a dumbbell in each hand, arms at your sides.

Action ❯ Step forward with your right leg, landing on your heel and then your forefoot. Lower your body by flexing the knee and hip of your front leg until the knee of your rear leg is almost in contact with the floor. Stand on the forward leg with the assistance of the rear leg. Lunge forward with the opposite leg. Do an equal number of repetitions on each leg.

Gina's Tip: Keep your torso upright during the lunge and make sure your leading knee is pointing in the same direction as the foot throughout the exercise. This exercise can also be done holding a medicine ball in front of you.

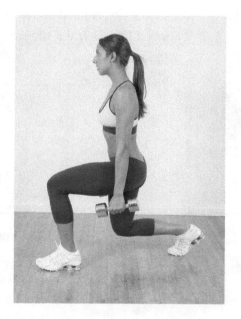 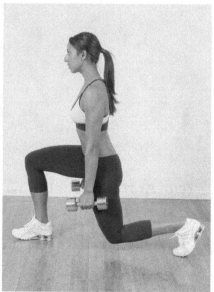

❯ **Dumbbell Step-Up on Bench or Step** (page 84)

❯ **Dumbbell Bench Press** (page 79)

Dumbbell Chest Fly on Ball

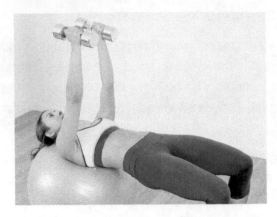

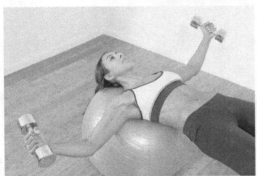

To start > Sit on a ball holding the dumbbells on your upper thighs. Kick the weights up to your shoulders and roll down, walking your feet out in front of you until your head and upper back are resting on the ball. Hold the dumbbells above your chest with your elbows slightly bent.

Action > Lower the dumbbells to your sides until your chest muscles are stretched. Bring the dumbbells together in a hugging motion until the dumbbells nearly touch.

Gina's Tip: Pretend you're hugging a big redwood tree. Only the shoulder joint is moving in this one.

Two-Arm Dumbbell Row

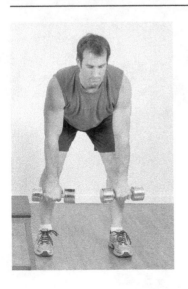

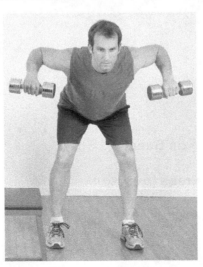

To start > Stand and bend at the waist at almost a 90-degree angle. Hold a dumbbell in each hand with your palms facing toward you.

Action > Lift the dumbbells up and next to your rib cage area. Return to the starting position.

Overhead Shoulder Press

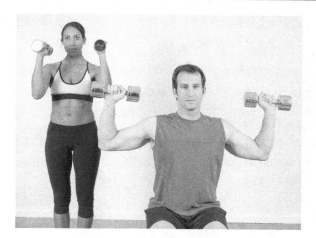

To start > Stand or sit with a dumbbell in each hand, elbows bent and wrists at shoulder level. Your palms should be facing in toward your ears if standing, facing forward if sitting. Your feet should be hip-width apart, with your knees in a soft position.

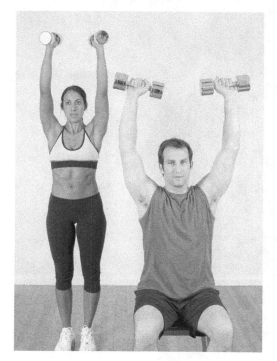

Action > Press the weights overhead until your elbows are nearly straight but not locked. Lower to the starting position.

Gina's Tip: If you experience shoulder discomfort, such as nerve impingement, it is best to use the arm position for the standing version.

Dumbbell Single-Arm Biceps Curl, Alternating Arms

To start > Stand with a dumbbell in each hand, arms at your sides with palms facing toward you and arms straight.

Action > Bend your elbows while rotating your forearms until your forearms are vertical and your palms are facing your shoulders. Lower your arms to the starting position.

Gina's Tip: When you become accustomed to this version you may substitute the Dumbbell Concentration Curl (page 118) for more of a challenge.

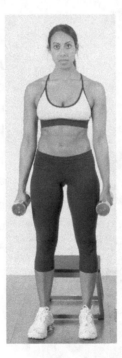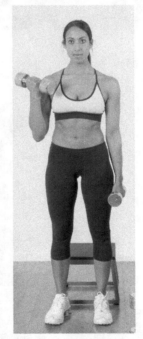

Lying Dumbbell Triceps Extension

To start > Sit on stability ball holding a dumbbell in each hand, close to your chest, then walk your feet forward until your head and upper back are supported on the ball. Your feet should be hip-width apart and flat on the floor. Keep your hips raised throughout the entire movement. Position the dumbbells over your head with your arms extended.

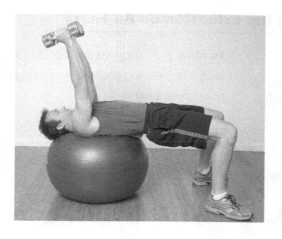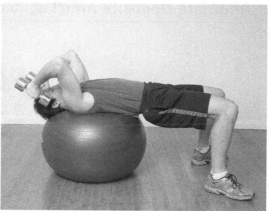

Action ❯ Lower the dumbbells by bending your elbows until the dumbbells are on either side of your head. Extend your arms.

Gina's Tip: Do not allow your shoulders to change position forward or back.

Figure Four

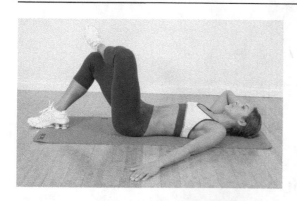

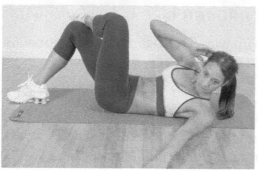

To start ❯ Lie on your back on a mat with your knees bent, feet flat on the floor. Place your right hand on your head, behind your ears. Rest your left ankle on your right knee. Place your left arm on the floor, palm down.

Action ❯ Slowly twist yourself forward as you bring your right elbow toward your left knee. Pause, then lower yourself and repeat for a set. Switch positions so that your right ankle lies across your left knee and repeat the move for another set.

Alternate Opposite Arm/Leg and Hip Extension on All Fours

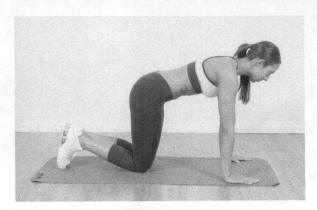

To start › Position yourself on all fours on a mat, keeping your neck in a neutral position as shown.

Action › Extend one leg behind you while extending the opposite arm in front of you, then pause and lower yourself to the starting position.

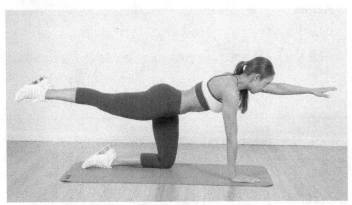

Workout with No Equipment

BEGINNER: WEEKS 1 THROUGH 6

- Warm up with 5 to 10 minutes of continuous cardio exercise, such as walking or stair-climbing.
- Do one set of 10 to 15 repetitions per exercise.
- Allow 1 to 2 minutes of rest between sets
- Train on three nonconsecutive days per week: Monday, Wednesday, Friday or Tuesday, Thursday, Saturday.

Squat with Arms at Sides

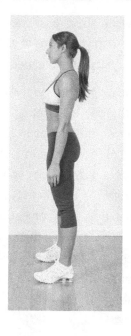

To start ❯ Stand with your feet parallel and shoulder-width apart, arms at your sides.

Action ❯ Bend your legs, keeping your back straight, and look slightly upward to keep your neck in alignment with your spine. Lower yourself until your thighs are parallel or almost parallel to the floor. Do not allow your knees to extend past your toes. Pause, then return to the starting position by pushing through the middle of your feet instead of your toes.

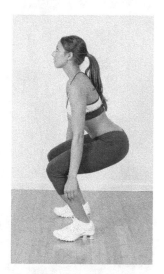

Gina's Tip: Act as if you are going to sit down on a chair and your body will automatically be in the right position.

Wall Push-Up

To start ❯ Stand in front of a wall with your feet hip-width apart and place your hands on the wall slightly wider than your shoulders. Move your feet back behind

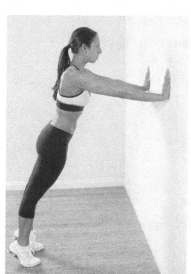

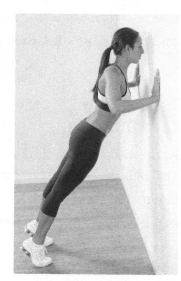

you so that you have room to lean into the wall.

Action ❯ Slowly lower your upper body toward the wall, being sure not to hit the wall with your head. (Sounds funny, but I've seen it happen.) Push off and return to the starting position.

Stationary Lunge

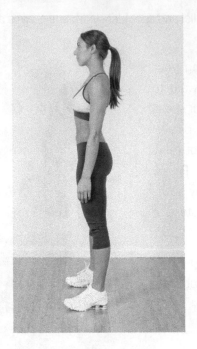

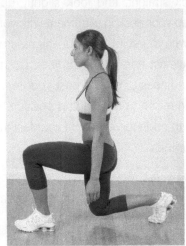

To start > Stand with your feet hip-width apart, your weight more on your heels than on your toes. Keep your arms at your sides, your stomach tucked in, and your shoulders squared.

Action > Step forward with your left foot about one stride. As your foot comes down, bend both knees until your left thigh is parallel to the floor (your right heel will come up). Step back to the standing position, then lunge forward with the right foot to finish a repetition.

> **Abdominal Crunch** (page 82)

> **Figure Four** (page 91)

> **Prone Back Extension with Hands on Lower Back** (page 82)

BEGINNER: WEEKS 7 THROUGH 12

- Warm up with 5 to 10 minutes of continuous cardio exercise, such as walking or stair-climbing.
- Do one to two sets of 10 to 15 repetitions per exercise.
- Allow 1 to 2 minutes of rest between sets.
- Train on three nonconsecutive days per week: Monday, Wednesday, Friday or Tuesday, Thursday, Saturday.

Squat with Arm Raise

To start ❯ Stand with your feet parallel and shoulder-width apart, arms at your sides.

Action ❯ Raise your arms straight out in front of you with palms facing down as shown. Bend your legs, keeping your back straight, and look slightly upward to protect your spine and neck. Lower yourself until your thighs are parallel to the floor. Do not allow your knees to extend past your toes. Pause, then return to the starting position by pushing through the middle of your feet.

Gina's Tip: Don't be tempted to go up on your toes or rock back on your heels, as you may lose your balance.

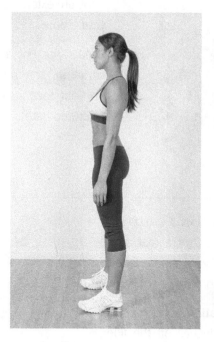 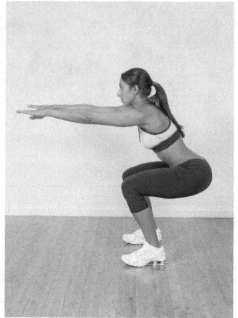

❯ **Stationary Lunge** (page 94)

Push-Up on Knees, on the Floor

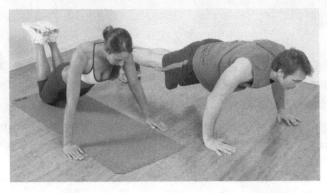

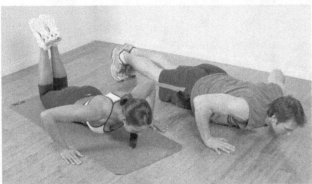

To start ❯ Position yourself with your palms on the floor, slightly more than shoulder-width apart, arms extended. Your knees are bent and on the floor; your lower legs are lifted up behind you.

Action ❯ Keeping your back straight, lower yourself toward the floor until your chest is close to the floor but not touching it. Then push up until your arms are extended again. Do not lock your elbows.

Gina's Tip: For a more challenging variation, try the military push-up on your toes instead of your knees (pictured here).

Reverse Crunch

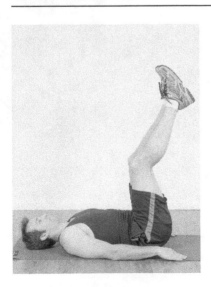

To start ❯ Lie on your back on a mat, arms at your sides. Extend your legs vertically.

Action ❯ Lift your hips 3 inches off the floor, pause, and lower them to the starting position.

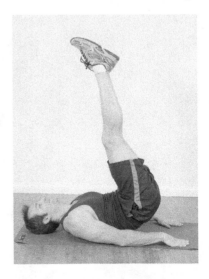

Bicycle

To start ❯ Lie on your back on a mat with your knees bent, feet off the floor, hands behind your head.

Action ❯ Leading with your right elbow, twist your torso up and toward the outside of your left knee. Immediately move toward the other side—left elbow toward the outside of the right knee.

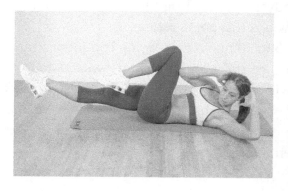 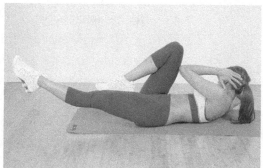

❯ **Figure Four** (page 91)

Prone Back Extension with Arms Straight in Front

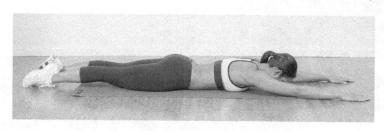

To start ❯ Lie facedown on a mat with your arms extended as shown.

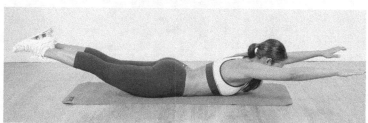

Action ❯ Lift your chest, head, and arms as well as your legs, extending your lower back. Be sure to keep your neck in line with your spine.

Machine Workouts

If you prefer to work out on machines either at home or at the gym, the following lower-body and upper-body machine exercises can be substituted for any of the lower-body/upper-body free-weight exercises described in the preceding pages. Both machines and free weights have their place in a sound exercise program, so use what's most convenient and comfortable for you. As a reminder, go back to chapter 3, reread the advantages and disadvantages of both, and decide what is best for you at this point in time.

Always warm up for 5 to 10 minutes by doing continuous cardio exercise such as walking or stair-climbing before weight training. Perform each exercise with good form, and stretch *after* your workout. Remember, when you use machines, select the weight (or load) that will allow you to perform the exercise in good form for the designated number of repetitions.

Leg Press

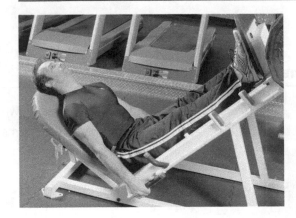

To start > Sit on the machine with your back against the support pad. Place your feet on the platform slightly more than hip-width apart. Push your legs out so that you can release the dock lever and grasp the handles at your sides.

Action > Lower the platform by flexing your hips and your knees until your knees are just short of complete flexion. Return to the starting position by extending your knees and hips.

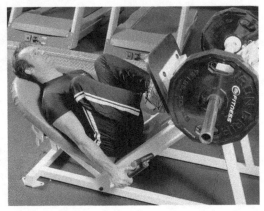

Gina's Tips: Adjust the platform safety brace and the back support to accommodate a full range of motion. Keep your knees pointed in the same direction as your feet throughout the movement, and don't allow your heels to raise off the platform; push with your entire foot.

Leg Extension

To start > Sit on the machine with your back against the support pad. Place your shins against the padded lever with your feet underneath the lever and your knees parallel to it. Hold the handles at your sides loosely for support.

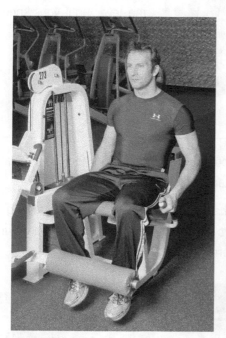

Action > Lift the lever up and forward by extending your knees until your legs are straight. Return to the starting position by bending your knees.

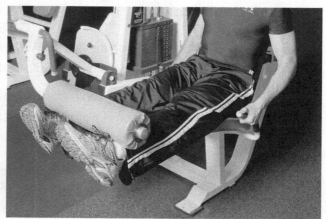

Gina's Tip: As you get into heavier weights on this, your stabilizer muscles will engage to keep you on the seat. If you continually come up off the seat, lower the weight.

Seated Leg Curl

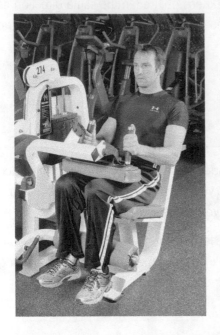

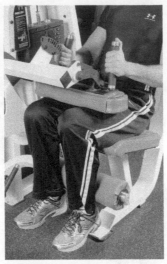

To start ❯ Sit on the machine with your back against the support pad. Place your calves on top of the padded lever. Adjust the lap pad so that it sits on thighs just above your knees. Grasp the handles on the lap support.

Action ❯ Pull the padded lever to the backs of your thighs by flexing your knees. Pause, then raise the lever until your knees are straight again.

Seated Cable Row

To start ❯ Sit on the machine with your knees bent and your feet on the platform in front of you. Grab the cable attachment handle.

Action ❯ Pull the cable attachment handle to your waist while maintaining a straight lower back. Pull your shoulders back and push your chest forward during the contraction. Return until your arms are extended.

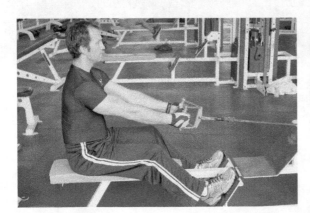

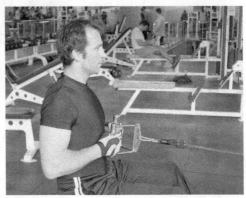

Assisted Pull-Up

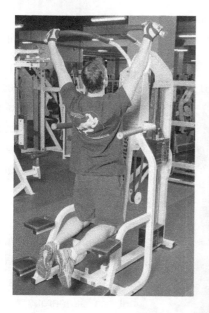

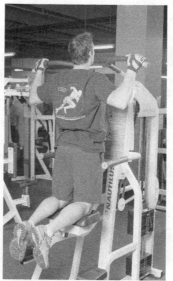

To start ❯ Grab the bar with a wide overhand grip and kneel on the assistance lever or platform.

Action ❯ Pull your body up until your neck reaches your hands, then lower yourself until your arms and shoulders are fully extended.

Gina's Tip: The more weight you choose, the easier this exercise gets. Be sure to challenge yourself.

Pull-Up Using Body Weight Only

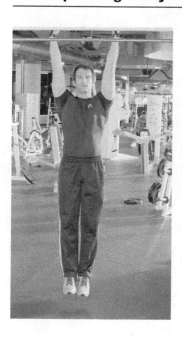

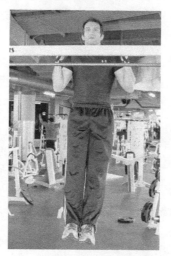

To start ❯ Grasp the handles on the pull-up bar firmly.

Action ❯ With your arms straight, hang from the bar and pull yourself up so that your chin is over the bar, with your hands nearly touching your chest. During your ascent, focus on contracting your lats, and be careful not to swing your body or lean too far backward. Lower yourself back to the starting position.

Gina's Tip: The narrower your grip, the more you work the lower lats during the exercise.

Lat Pull-Down

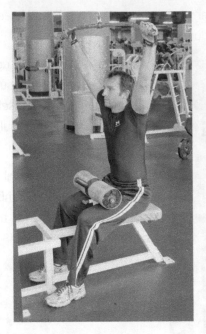

To start > Sit on the machine with thighs firmly under the support pads. Grab the cable bar with a wide overhand grip.

Action > Pull the cable bar down to your upper chest while slightly leaning back into a 45-degree angle. Touch your chest

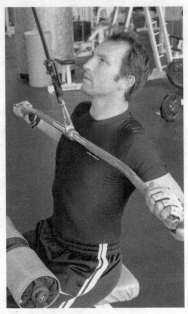

with the bar, but do not bang the bar on your sternum. Return until your arms and shoulders are fully extended.

Gina's Tip: Under no circumstances should you pull the cable bar down behind your neck. This is not only dangerous if the cable happens to break, but it also adds stress to the cervical spine.

Machine Chest Fly

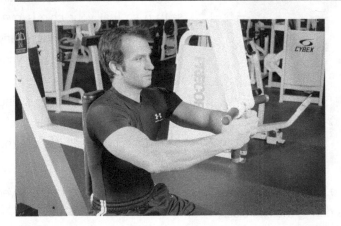

To start > Sit on the machine with your back against the pad and your feet on the floor. Grasp the machine's handles with both hands while your arms are extended at shoulder height.

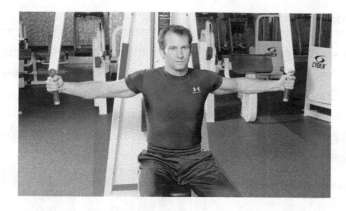

Action ❯ Slowly pull each handle toward the midline of your body until your hands nearly touch each other. Then slowly return to the starting position to complete one repetition. Your back should remain in contact with the pad and your arms should stay at chest level while performing this exercise.

Machine Overhead Press

To start ❯ Adjust the seat height so that the handles or bars are about even with your shoulders. Sit on the machine with your back against the seat and your feet flat on the floor or firmly on a foot bar, if there is one.

Action ❯ Grasp the handles and press the weight upward smoothly and slowly until your arms are extended but not locked. Lower the weight back to shoulder height, without allowing the lifted weight to rest on the weight stack. Be sure to breath—exhale on the lift; inhale while bringing the weight down.

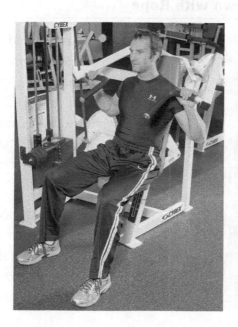 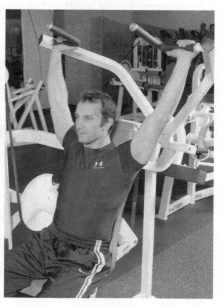

Machine Triceps Extension

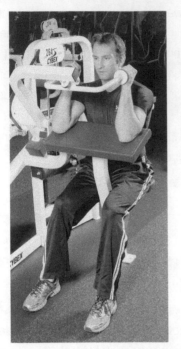

To start › Adjust the pad to support your chest. Sit on the machine with your chest against the pad and bring the handles up. Grasp the handles with your palms facing each other and your arms parallel to each other, resting the backs of your arms on the support pad. Maintain a straight back by pushing your hips toward the back of the seat.

Action › With your arms parallel to each other and keeping your shoulders from rising, exhale while pushing the handles down and away from you. Push until your arms are straight, then inhale as you slowly return to the starting position.

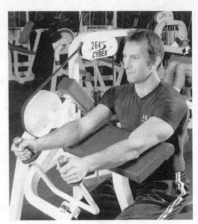

Machine Triceps Push-Down with Rope

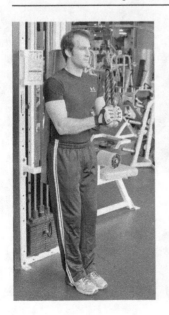
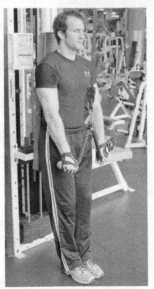

To start › Stand with your back against the support pad, facing away from the machine, knees in a soft position and feet together. Grab the rope with both hands at the bottom where the grip balls sit. Your forearms should be parallel to the floor, elbows pulled in toward your body.

Action › Push down and outward with the rope as you extend your elbows, keeping a slight bend in your elbows at the end of the movement instead of locking them.

Dip

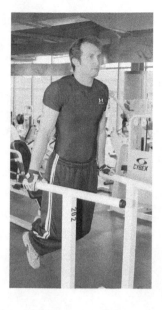 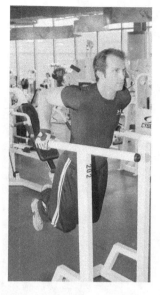

To start ❯ Position yourself on the bars with your arms straight and your elbows locked, with a "knuckles out" grip. Bend the knees and cross your ankles. Keep your wrists straight. Keep your chest out and your shoulders pulled back.

Action ❯ Bend your elbows and lower yourself until you feel the stretch across your chest, then press up and exhale.

Machine Biceps Curl

To start ❯ Adjust the seat height so that your fulcrum (moving joint) is about even with your elbows. Sit with your chest against the support pad and your feet flat on the floor.

Action ❯ Place your elbows on the support pad, grasp the handles in an extended elbow position, then curl the bar in toward you by bending your elbows. Pause and lower your arms to the starting position.

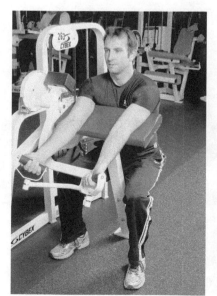 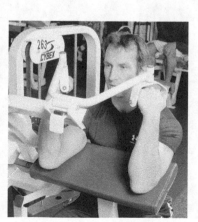

Machine Lower-Back Extension

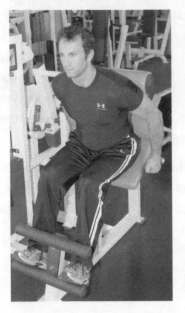 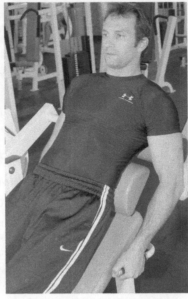

To start › Since machines vary from gym to gym, adjust your position according to the guidelines posted on the machine itself.

Action › Grasp the handles and slowly extend your torso in a slow, controlled motion, your back making contact with the lumbar pad. Pause and return to the starting position.

Machine Abdominal Crunch

To start › Sit on the machine and rest your shins under the support rollers. Place your elbows on the support pads and grasp the handles. Keep your elbows tucked slightly in toward your body.

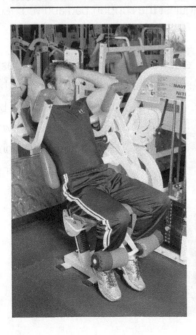 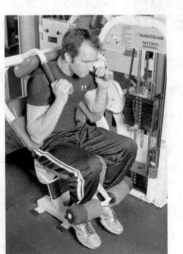

Action › Keeping your neck in a neutral position, crunch with your abs while pulling down on the handles. Pause and return to the starting position.

Incline Reverse Crunch

To start ❯ Lie on your back on an incline bench with your head at the top of the incline. Reaching up, grasp the pads above your head.

Action ❯ With your knees slightly bent, raise your legs and then your hips until they are perpendicular to the floor.

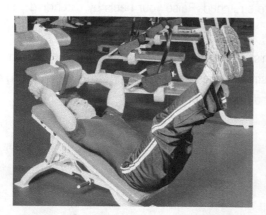
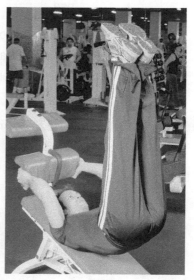

Decline Twisting Crunch with Medicine Ball

To start ❯ Set the ball next to a decline ab bench and lie on the bench as shown, with your feet secure under the foam rollers.

Action ❯ Grab the ball from the floor and, holding it close to your chest with your torso at a 45-degree angle, twist from right to left.

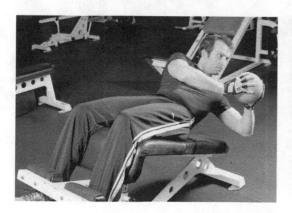
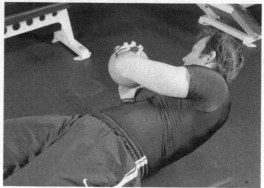

Seated Calf Raise

To start > Sit on the machine and place your toes on the lower part of the platform with your heels extending off. Position your lower thighs under the lever pad.

Action > Hold the handles and lift the lever slightly by pushing your heels up, then release the support lever. Lower your heels by bending your ankles until your calves are stretched. Raise your heels by extending your ankles as high as possible.

Gina's Tip: This can be done while pushing through the big toes, keeping your feet pointing straight ahead, or by turning your toes outward or inward. Be sure to maintain good upper-body posture.

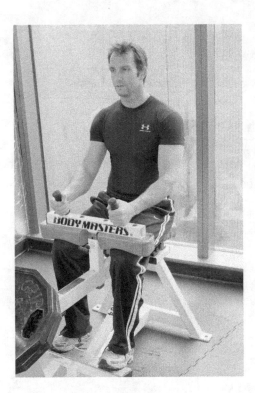
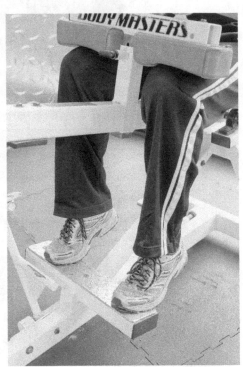

Make It Harder

Beginners, intermediates, and advanced exercisers: Want to make your current workout more challenging? Add in cardio intervals of 1 to 3 minutes between 8 to 12 repetitions of various exercises and move quickly to and from each one in a circuit-type fashion. This will feel more challenging, increase your heart rate, make your workout more fun and time efficient, and burn more overall calories!

Example:

Warm up by walking on the treadmill for 5 minutes

Dumbbell Squat

Treadmill walking, 2 minutes at a moderate pace

Stability Ball Leg Curl

Treadmill walking, 2 minutes at a moderate pace

Dumbbell Bench Press

Treadmill walking, 2 minutes at a moderate pace

Dumbbell One-Arm Row

Treadmill walking, 2 minutes at a moderate pace

Dumbbell Biceps Curl

Stair-climbing machine, 2 minutes at a moderate pace

Dumbbell Triceps Kickback

Stair-climbing machine, 2 minutes at a moderate pace

Abdominal Crunch

Stair-climbing machine, 2 minutes at a moderate pace

Prone Back Extension with Hands on Lower Back

Stretch

Intermediate Workouts

If you consider yourself an intermediate exerciser, you will follow this workout for twelve weeks, including the progressive variations. If you need more of a challenge, you can add advanced exercises from the lists beginning on page 127.

Cardio

INTERMEDIATE: WEEKS 1 THROUGH 12

- Do cardio five times per week; your total workout time, including warm-up and cooldown, should be 30 minutes on weight-training days, 40 minutes on non-weight-training days.

- On weight-training days, do your 20 minutes of intervals immediately following weight training.

INTERVALS FOR INTERMEDIATE: WEEKS 1 THROUGH 6

- Warm up for 5 minutes at a 55 to 75 percent HR max.
- Do 1 minute at 80 to 85 percent HR max, followed by 2 minutes of active recovery at 55 to 75 percent HR max; repeat for 20 to 30 minutes.
- Cool down for 5 minutes.

INTERVALS FOR INTERMEDIATE: WEEKS 7 THROUGH 12

- Warm up for 5 minutes at a 55 to 75 percent HR max.
- Do 2 minutes at 80 to 85 percent HR max, followed by 2 minutes of active recovery at 55 to 75 percent HR max; repeat for 20 to 30 minutes.
- Cool down for 5 minutes.

Fit Tips for Intermediates

Follow these suggestions for a better workout:

- At this stage you can vary the environment in which you do your exercises to stave off boredom.
- Because your goal is fat loss and general fitness, the set and rep scheme is geared toward that. If at any time you change your goal to, say, build strength or put on more muscle, the set and rep scheme would change. For example, lower reps (6 to 8) and heavier loads to build strength, increased volume (more sets) to add bulk.
- Take the time to look at the pictures and read the exercise descriptions to ensure proper technique.
- Always warm up for at least 5 minutes prior to weight training. For best results, stretch at the end of your session.
- Choose weights that allow you to handle the designated number of repetitions with good form.
- Follow the weekly progressions as outlined in the intermediate workout lists.
- Take the rest periods of 2 to 3 minutes between sets and exercises. The harder you train, the longer rest periods you may need, so don't be afraid to rest for up to 4 minutes between sets if you need to.
- Perform each exercise in a smooth manner and through a full range of motion.
- Take note that in this phase of training, the order of some of the exercises is different than in the beginner programs. This is done to give certain muscles a chance to rest before hitting them again in the same workout.
- The no equipment workouts can be very strenuous! Don't do them every day. Do your cardio on alternating days instead.

Weight Training

INTERMEDIATE WEEKS 1 THROUGH 4

- Warm up with 5 to 10 minutes of continuous cardio exercise, such as walking or stair-climbing.
- Do three sets of 8 to 10 repetitions per exercise.
- Allow 1 to 2 minutes of rest between sets.
- Train on three nonconsecutive days per week: Monday, Wednesday, Friday or Tuesday, Thursday, Saturday.

> **Dumbbell Squat** (page 78)

> **Dumbbell Bench Press** (page 79)

Dumbbell Pull-Over on Stability Ball

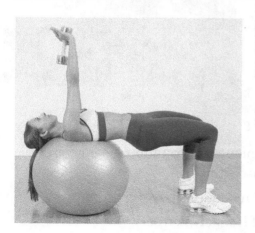 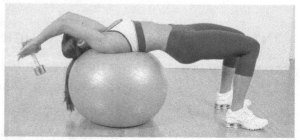

To start › Rest your head, shoulders, and upper back on the ball, with your feet firmly on the floor. Grab hold of the dumbbell with both hands as shown.

Action › As you inhale, bring your arms straight up above your chest, holding the weight firmly. As you bend your elbows, lower the weight behind your head until you feel the stretch in your chest and arms. Exhale as you return to the starting position.

> **Overhead Shoulder Press** (page 89)

> **Stability Ball Leg Curl** (page 79)

> **Dumbbell Biceps Curl** (page 81)

> **Lying Dumbbell Triceps Extension** (page 90)

> **Prone Back Extension with Arms Straight in Front** (page 97)

Abdominal Crunch on Stability Ball

To start ❯ Sit on the ball with your feet firmly on the floor about hip-width apart.

Action ❯ Walk your feet forward, rolling your torso down until your thighs and torso are parallel to the floor. With your fingertips by your ears, curl up into an abdominal crunch.

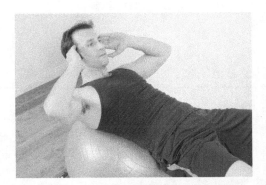 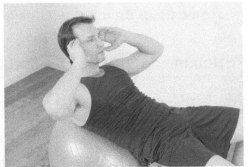

INTERMEDIATE: WEEKS 5 THROUGH 8

- Warm up with 5 to 10 minutes of continuous cardio exercise, such as walking or stair-climbing.
- Do three sets of 8 to 10 repetitions per exercise.
- Allow 1 to 2 minutes of rest between sets.
- Train on three nonconsecutive days per week: Monday, Wednesday, Friday or Tuesday, Thursday, Saturday.

Dumbbell Squat Jump

To start ❯ Stand with a dumbbell in each hand. Look straight ahead, keeping your back straight, your arms straight at your sides, and your feet flat on the floor, with your weight equally distributed between your forefoot and your heel. Your knees should point in the same direction as your feet throughout the movement.

Action > Lower your-self into the squat, then forcefully jump up as high as you can, continuing to keep your arms straight, so that your feet are off the floor. Land in a "soft" knee position, *never* with your knees locked and straight.

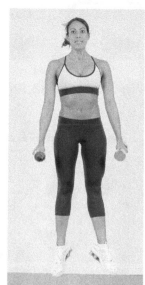

> **Dumbbell Chest Fly on Ball** (page 88)

> **Dumbbell One-Arm Row** (page 80)

> **Dumbbell Lateral Raise** (page 85)

Good Morning

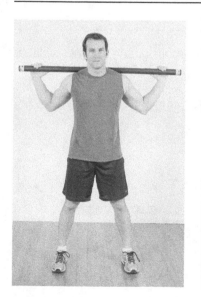

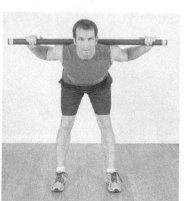

To start > Stand and place a barbell or a body bar across your shoulders. Your knees should be slightly bent.

Action > Bend at the hips, keeping your lower back arched. Lower your upper body until it is roughly parallel to the floor, or until you can't maintain the lower back arch. Then stand back up following the same path.

Gina's Tip: Do not lock or hyperextend the knees. Also, do not round your lower back. These are the two most common mistakes. This exercise can be dangerous if performed incorrectly, so take good care or skip it.

> **Dumbbell Single-Arm Biceps Curl, Alternating Arms** (page 90)

Seated One-Arm Overhead Triceps Extension

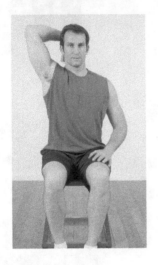 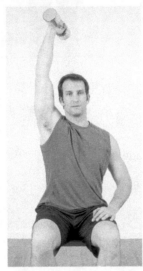

To start > Sit on a bench with your feet flat on the floor. Holding a dumbbell, bring your right arm up by the side of your head with your elbow bent, keeping the dumbbell behind your head.

Action > Inhale and then exhale as you straighten (or extend) your elbow above your head. Lower your arm slowly to the starting position. Alternate arms.

Back Extension on Stability Ball

To start > Lie facedown on the ball with your toes on the floor hip-width apart and your hands on your lower back as shown.

Action > Extend your lower back by raising your chest and head. Pause, then lower yourself to the starting position.

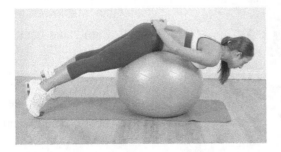 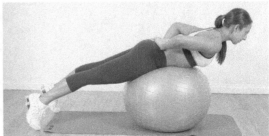

Weighted Abdominal Crunch and Reach

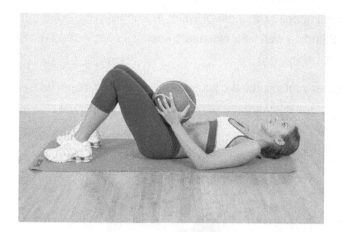

To start > Lie on your back with your knees bent, feet on the floor hip-width apart.

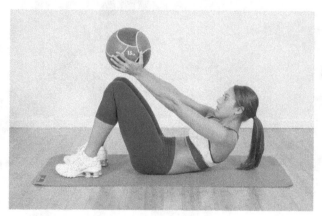

Action > Holding a medicine ball (or a dumbbell) in front of you, reach toward your knees while doing a traditional ab crunch, then return to the starting position.

INTERMEDIATE: WEEKS 9 THROUGH 12

- Warm up with 5 to 10 minutes of continuous cardio exercise, such as walking or stair-climbing.
- Do three sets of 8 to 10 repetitions per exercise.
- Allow 1 to 2 minutes of rest between sets.
- Train on three nonconsecutive days per week: Monday, Wednesday, Friday or Tuesday, Thursday, Saturday.

> Dumbbell Walking Lunge (page 87)

One-Leg Squat with Forward Reach

To start > Place a dumbbell or a bottle of water in front of your leg about an arm's length away. Standing with your feet apart, keep your left foot on the floor and lift your right foot behind you.

Action > As you lower yourself into the squat with your left leg, reach with both arms toward the object. This is not a full squat.

Gina's Tip: Do this in front of a mirror so that you don't have to look down toward the object, which could cause you to lose balance and form.

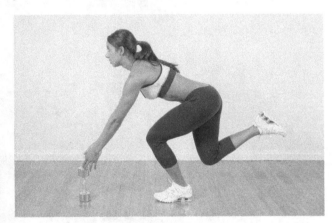

Push-Up with T Roll

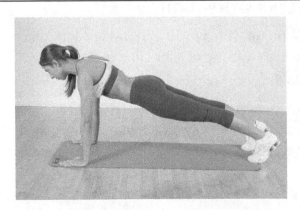

To start > Position yourself with your palms on the floor, slightly more than shoulder-width apart, arms extended. Your legs should be straight out behind you; balance on your toes.

Action ❯ Keeping your back straight, lower yourself toward the floor until your chest is close to the floor but not touching it. Then push up until your arms are extended again and bring your left arm up straight toward the ceiling, creating the letter T with your upper body. Return to the starting position.

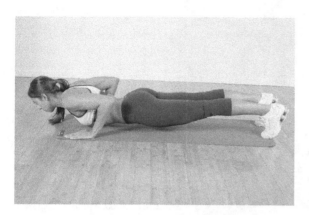 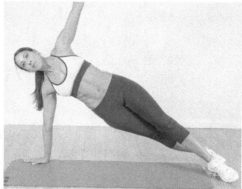

Facedown Dumbbell Row on Stability Ball

To start ❯ Place a dumbbell on either side of the ball. Lie on your stomach on the ball with your toes placed firmly on the floor and your knees bent. Keep your neck in a neutral position.

Action ❯ Holding a dumbbell in each hand, pull both weights straight up to your sides, elbows toward the ceiling. Exhale on the way up.

Return your arms slowly to the floor.

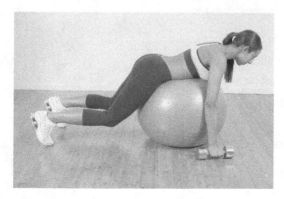 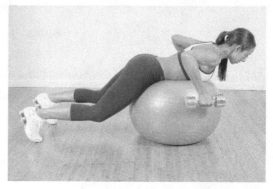

Dumbbell Front Raise and Lateral Raise—combine both for 10 reps each (See page 85 for Dumbbell Lateral Raise)

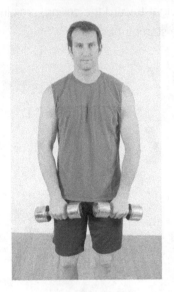
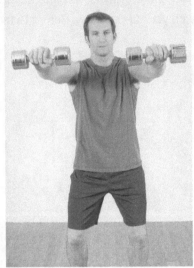

To start > Stand with a dumbbell in each hand, hands in front of your waist, palms down. Your feet should be hip-width apart, with your knees slightly bent and your shoulders pulled back.

Action > Raise both arms with your elbows fixed in a 10- to 30-degree angle throughout until your upper arm is parallel to the floor. Lower to the starting position.

> Good Morning (page 113)

Dumbbell Concentration Curl

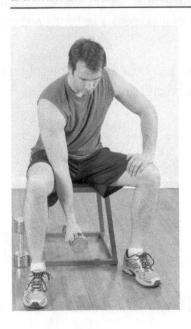

To start > Sit on a bench. Hold a dumbbell in your right hand. Place the back of your upper arm on the inner thigh of the same side leg. Lean into the leg to raise your elbow slightly.

Action > Bend your elbow to raise the dumbbell to the front of your shoulder. Lower the dumbbell until your arm is fully extended. Complete all reps on this side, then switch arms.

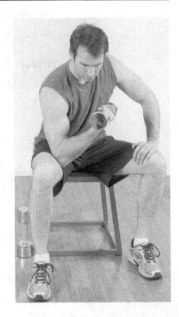

❯ Dumbbell Triceps Kickback (page 81)

Weighted Back Extension on Stability Ball

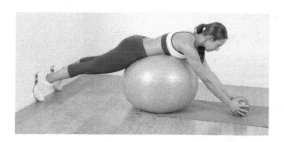

To start ❯ Lie facedown on the ball, with your feet anchored against the wall, hip-width apart and your arms extended in front holding a medicine ball as shown.

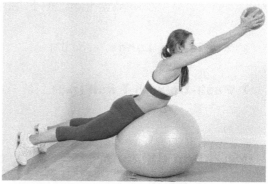

Action ❯ Extend your lower back by raising your chest, head, and arms. Pause, then lower yourself to the starting position.

Weighted Lateral Crunch on Stability Ball

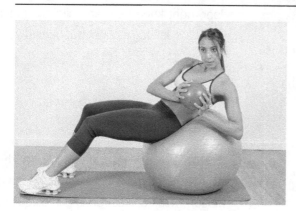

To start ❯ Sit on the ball at a 45-degree angle with your feet firmly on the floor and your abs in. Hold a medicine ball at chest level and squeeze to contract the chest.

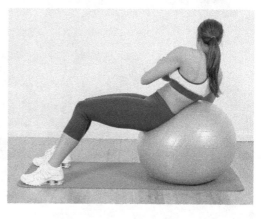

Action ❯ While continuing to squeeze the medicine ball, slowly twist to the left, then to the right, alternating sides continually for one set.

Workout with No Equipment

INTERMEDIATE: WEEKS 1 THROUGH 6

- Warm up with 5 to 10 minutes of continuous cardio exercise, such as walking or stair-climbing.
- Do two sets of 10 to 12 repetitions per exercise.
- Allow 1 to 2 minutes of rest between sets.
- Train on three nonconsecutive days per week: Monday, Wednesday, Friday or Tuesday, Thursday, Saturday.

> **Stationary Lunge** (page 94)

> **Push-Up with T Roll** (page 116)

Mountain Climber

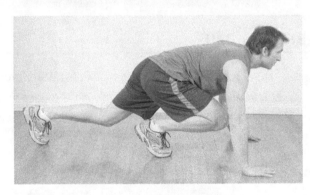

To start › Stand as if you are on a starting block for a footrace: hands on the floor, right knee bent and slightly under your hips, left leg straight out behind you.

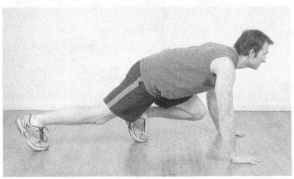

Action › Keeping your hands on the floor, switch leg positions with a hopping motion. Think of it as running in place but with your hands on the floor. Moving each leg forward once counts as 1 rep.

Pike Press

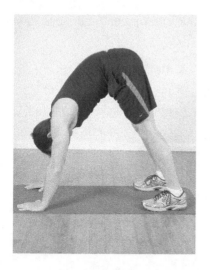

To start › Position yourself with your feet hip-width apart and your hands on the floor under your shoulders. Walk your hands in toward your feet until your body is in a V shape as shown.

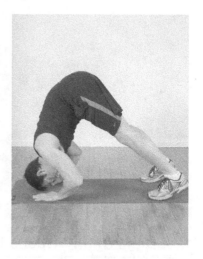

Action › Lower yourself into a push-up, keeping your head and neck in line with your spine, until you feel the top of your head slightly touch the floor. Push back up to the starting position.

Gina's Tip: For an equally challenging variation intermediate and advanced exercisers can try the Diamond Push-Up (page 132).

One-Leg Squat Jump

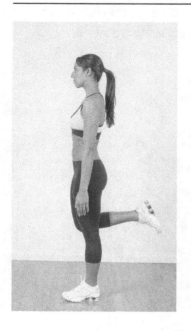

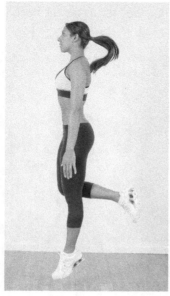

To start › Standing with your feet apart, begin with your left foot on the floor and your right foot lifted and back behind you.

Action › Lower yourself into a squat with your left leg, your arms at your sides, then forcefully jump up as high as you comfortably can, landing in a bent, or "soft," knee position.

Plank

To start > Lie facedown on a mat with your elbows bent and close to your chest, and your hands in fists.

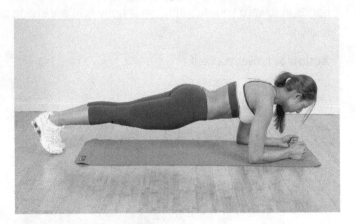

Action > Push up off the floor, rising onto your toes and elbows. Keep your back flat. Contract your abs and hold for 30 to 90 seconds, then lower yourself to the starting position.

Bench/Chair Triceps Dip

To start > Place your hands on the edge of a bench, heels together on the floor.

Action > Lower your body until it is fully stretched or until your rear end nearly touches the floor, then raise yourself back to the starting position.

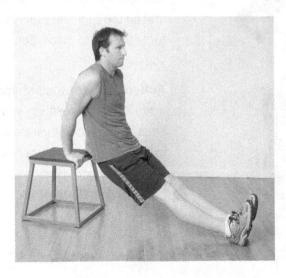
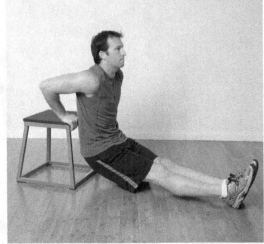

Lying Side Crunch

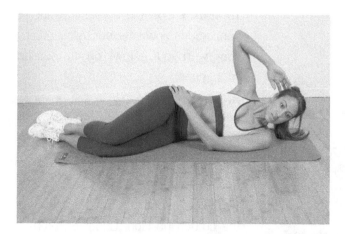

To start > Lie on your left side on a mat with both legs together, knees and hips bent. Place your right hand on your head and your left arm on the floor in front of you with your hand on the opposite hip.

Action > Crunch straight up to the side to work the side abdominal muscles (obliques). Repeat for a set then turn to the other side.

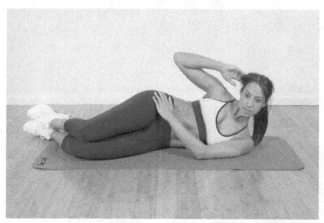

INTERMEDIATE: WEEKS 7 THROUGH 12

- Warm up with 5 to 10 minutes of continuous cardio exercise, such as walking or stair-climbing.
- Do three sets of 12 repetitions per exercise.
- Allow 1 to 2 minutes of rest between sets.
- Train on three nonconsecutive days per week: Monday, Wednesday, Friday or Tuesday, Thursday, Saturday.

Six-Count Bodybuilder

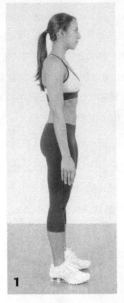

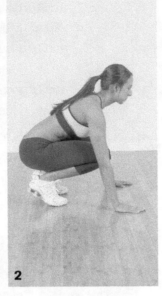

To start ❯ Count 1: from a standing position, crouch down so your palms touch the floor, with your elbows on the outside of your knees.

Action ❯ Count 2: in one movement, push off with your hands, legs and back straight behind you, into the "up" position of a push-up. Count 3: do a full push-up, going down for a count of three. Count 4: push up for the count of four. Count 5: jump back to the crouch position. Count 6: return to a standing position. That's 1 repetition.

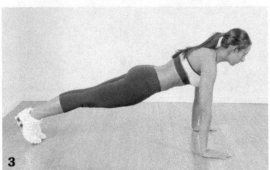

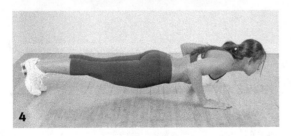

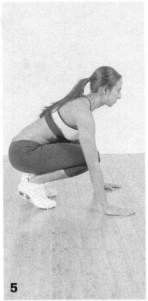

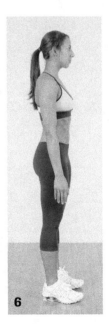

❯ **Push-Up with T Roll** (page 116)

❯ **Mountain Climber** (page 120)

❯ **Pike Press** (page 121)

Walking Lunge

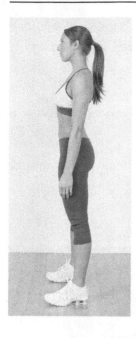

To start ❯ Stand with your arms at your sides.

Action ❯ Step forward with your right leg, landing on your heel and then your forefoot. Lower your body by flexing the knee and hip of your front leg until the knee of your rear leg is almost in contact with the floor.

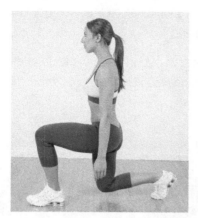

Stand on your forward leg with the assistance of the rear leg. Lunge forward with the opposite leg. Continue this walking motion by alternating lunges with opposite leg.

Gina's Tip: Keep your torso upright during the lunge phase and make sure your leading knee is pointing in the same direction as the foot throughout the exercise.

Bench/Chair Triceps Dip with Legs Elevated

To start ❯ Place your hands on the edge of a bench with your feet elevated on an adjacent bench.

Action ❯ Lower your body until it is fully stretched or until your rear end nearly touches the floor. Raise yourself back to the starting position.

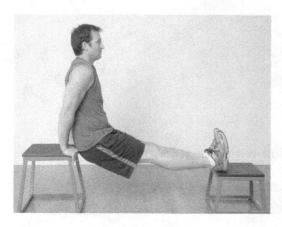 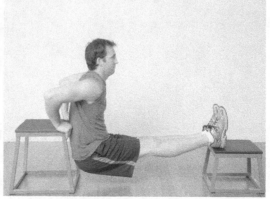

Crunch with Toe Reach, Legs at 45 degrees

To start > Lie on your back on a mat with your legs in the air at a 45-degree angle. Extend your arms straight up in the air. Your hips, back, and shoulders should all be touching the floor.

Action > Contract your abdominal muscles as you reach for your toes. Your back and shoulders should rise off the floor. Hold the position for a second, then slowly lower yourself.

Gina's Tip: Do not round your shoulders in an attempt to reach your toes. Keep your legs and toes pointed at a 45-degree angle throughout the exercise.

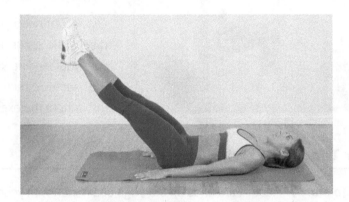

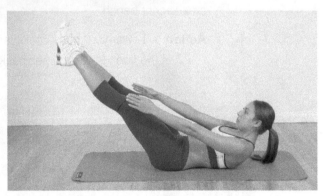

> **Prone Back Extension with Arms Straight in Front** (page 97)

> **Lying Side Crunch** (page 123)

Take It Up a Notch: For Advanced Exercisers

If you're able to perform the intermediate exercises with good form for the designated number of repetitions and sets, and/or you need a cardio boost, follow the instructions in this section for a more challenging workout.

Cardio

ADVANCED: WEEKS 1 THROUGH 12

- Warm up for 5 minutes.
- Do intervals. For weeks 1 through 6, do 3 minutes at 80 to 90 percent HR max, followed by 2 minutes of active recovery at 60 to 75 percent HR max; repeat for 20 to 40 minutes. For weeks 7 through 12, do 4 minutes at 80 to 90 percent HR max, then follow through the sequence as in weeks 1 through 6.
- Cool down for 5 minutes.
- Do cardio five times per week, for 20 minutes immediately following weight training or for 40 minutes on opposite days.
- Total workout time, including warm-up and cooldown: 30 minutes on weight-training days, 50 minutes on non-weight-training days.

Weight Training

In addition to the exercises you have already learned in the beginner and intermediate programs, you can add or substitute the following exercises to take yourself to a new level of fitness.

- Do three sets of 10 to 12 repetitions per exercise
- Allow 1 to 2 minutes of rest between sets
- Train on three nonconsecutive days per week: Monday, Wednesday, Friday or Tuesday, Thursday, Saturday.

Split Jump

To start > Stand with a dumbbell in each hand, arms at your sides.

Action > Step forward with your right leg, landing on your heel and then your forefoot. Lower your body by flexing the knee and hip of your front leg until the knee of the rear leg is almost in contact with the floor. Then forcefully jump up and switch feet in midair, landing on the opposite foot in a lunge.

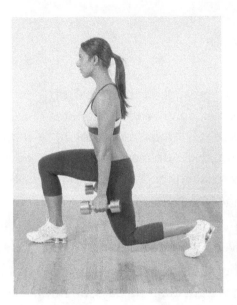 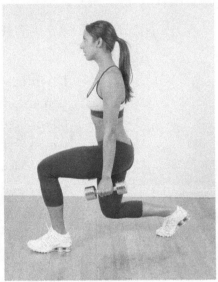

Elevated Leg Plank, Alternating Legs

To start > Lie facedown on a mat with your elbows bent and close to your chest and your hands in fists.

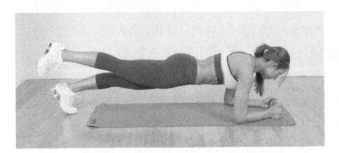

Action > Push up off the floor, rising onto your toes and elbows. Keep your back flat. Now raise your right leg, keeping your knee straight, just above the opposite leg. Contract your abs and hold for 30 to 90 seconds. Then lower and repeat with your left leg.

Lateral Box Jump-Over

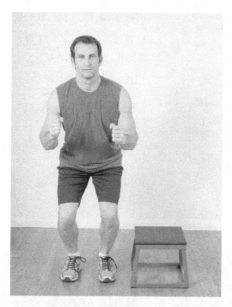

To start > Stand with your feet directly underneath you and your hands at chest level.

Action > Jump up sideways over the box, landing with your hands and feet directly underneath you. Immediately jump sideways back to the starting position. Repeat without pausing between the landing phases.

Gina's Tips: Explosively swinging your arms up helps with jump height. Avoid tucking your legs instead of truly jumping. Don't hunch; keep the chest up.

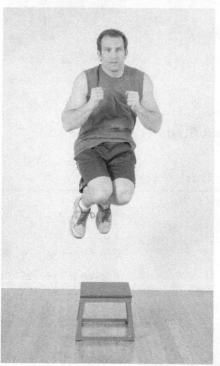

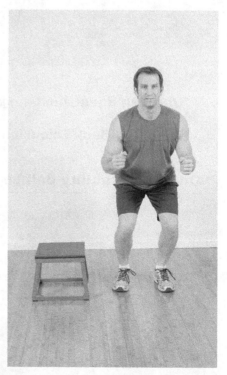

Flutter Kick

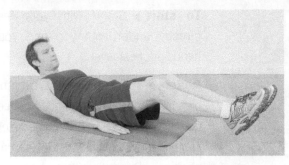

To start > Lie on your back with your hands slightly under your buttocks. Raise your upper body off the floor, keeping your chin slightly tucked to support your neck.

Action > Kick your legs up and down between 6 and 36 inches of the floor. Count 1, 2, 3, 1 and that equals 1 rep.

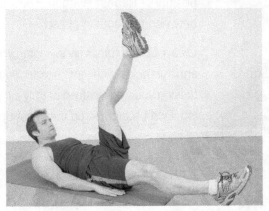

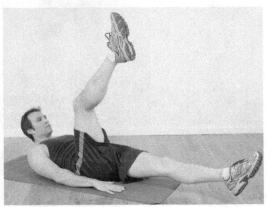

> **One-Leg Squat Jump** (page 121)

> **Weighted Back Extension on Stability Ball** (page 119)

One-Leg Stability Ball Leg Curl

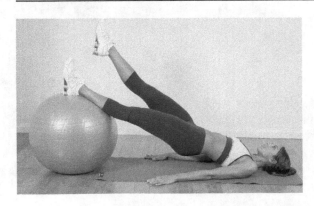

To start > Lie on your back on a mat. Place the ball under your left calf. Extend your right leg up into the air at a 45-degree angle. Raise your hips into the air as you push down into the ball with your left heel. At the top of the lift your body should be straight at a 30-degree angle to the floor. Hold the position.

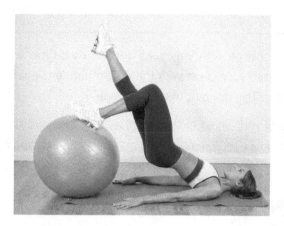

Action > Pull the ball in toward your glutes with your left leg, keeping your hips off the floor and keeping the other leg vertical. Bring the ball in as far as possible, then slowly release it back to the starting position.

Atomic Sit-Up

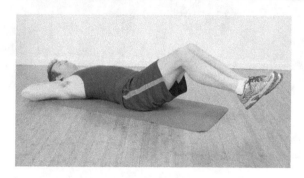

To start > Lie on your back with your hands behind your head. Extend your legs about 6 inches off the floor, with your knees slightly bent.

Action > Perform a sit-up while pulling your knees into your chest. Keeping your balance will be a challenge on this one.

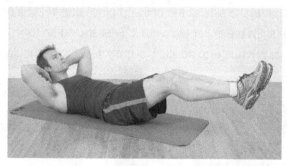

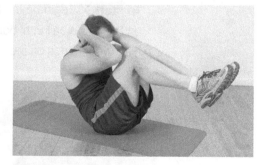

> **Incline Reverse Crunch** (page 107)

> **Pull-Up Using Body Weight Only** (page 101)

> **Decline Twisting Crunch with Medicine Ball** (page 107)

Diamond Push-Up

To start > Start in push-up position with your toes and hands on the floor, hands close together underneath your chest with the thumb and forefinger of each hand touching each other. This makes a diamond shape.

Action > Lower yourself until your chest almost touches the floor, and then push yourself back up, taking in a deep breath as you go down and exhaling as you push yourself back up.

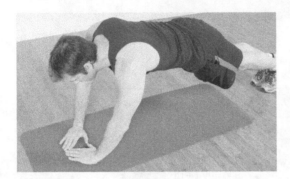 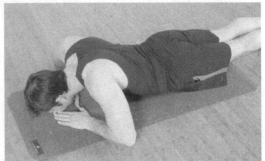

Jackknife on Stability Ball

To start > Begin on the floor at the side of the ball and place one leg at a time on top of the ball until both shins are in contact with it. Feet should be together. Place your hands on the floor in a push-up position, slightly wider than shoulder-width apart.

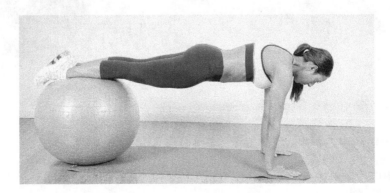

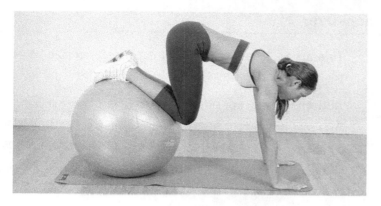

Action › Slowly pull your knees in toward your chest, then roll back out to starting position by retracing the path you followed for the inward motion.

› Elevated Leg Plank, Alternating Legs (page 128)

Advanced Stability Ball Push-Up

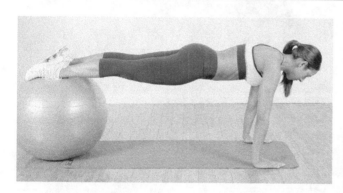

To start › Begin on the floor at the side of the ball and place one leg at a time on top of the ball until both shins are in contact with it. Your feet should be together. Place your hands on the floor in a push-up position, slightly wider than shoulder-width apart, with your wrists directly underneath your shoulders.

Action › Roll forward, placing your body weight on your hands, until the ball rests under your feet. Your body should be extended in a straight line from the ball. Keep your abdominal muscles tight and your body straight from your shoulders to your toes. Return to the starting position.

Gina's Tip: For increased difficulty, roll the ball back so that only your tiptoes are resting on it.

Lateral Foam Roll Jump-Over

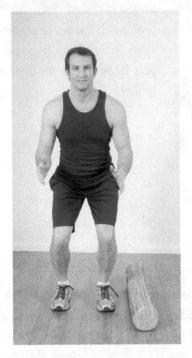

To start > Stand with your feet directly underneath you and your hands at chest level.

Action > Jump up sideways over the foam roll, landing with your feet directly underneath you. Immediately jump sideways back to the starting position. Repeat without pausing between the landing phases.

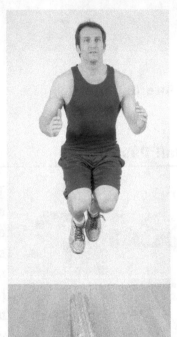

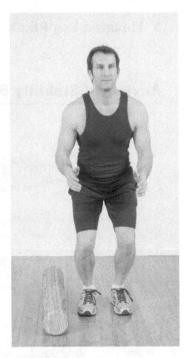

Gina's Tip: Explosively swinging your arms up helps with jump height.

Fine-Tuning the Food Formula: What to Do If You Want to Lose More

If you are eating all your meals and therefore all your daily calories, that's great. Do not, I repeat do *not* eat less. This will not help you lose more weight. Instead, either add exercise or increase the intensity of the exercise you are currently doing. To do this, choose one of the more difficult workouts if you are up to it. Or increase the intensity of your cardio by walking hills instead of flats; increasing the incline on the treadmill, stair-climber, or elliptical machine; or doing an interval program. But be sure to do only what you can handle.

Take It Up One More Notch with Peripheral Heart Action (PHA) Training

Peripheral Heart Action Training is a variation of circuit training designed to work your cardiovascular system by alternating lower-body exercises with upper-body exercises. This forces the heart to work harder by having to shunt blood up and down the body to the working muscles. It differs from traditional circuit training because you will use moderate to heavy weights instead of lighter weights during a circuit. It can also be done with body weight only to create an amazing cardiovascular and strength workout. The benefits? You'll maximize fat burning and increase postexercise oxygen consumption. You will also get maximum cardiovascular and muscular endurance by keeping blood moving from one body part to the next, not allowing it to pool in any one place for a period of time. Here's how you do it: Take your current workout and order the exercises so that you have a leg or ab/lower-back exercise followed by an upper-body exercise. Repeat this technique with three sequences of four to six exercises. Do between 8 to 20 repetitions with no rest between exercises. You can rest for up to 3 minutes between sequences. The workout would look like this:

Sequence #1
- Dumbbell Squat: 10 to 20 reps
- Abdominal Crunch: 10 to 20 reps
- Push-Up: 10 to 20 reps
- Prone Back Extension with Arms Straight in Front: 10 to 20 reps
- Figure Four: 10 to 20 reps
- Dumbbell Pull-Over on Stability Ball: 10 to 20 reps

Perform the routine one to three times through depending on your fitness level, then move on to the next sequence.

Sequence #2
- Dumbbell Squat Jump: 10 to 20 reps
- Pike Press: 10 to 20 reps
- Leg Press: 10 to 20 reps
- Push-Up with T Roll: 10 to 20 reps
- Machine Abdominal Crunch: 10 to 20 reps

Perform the routine one to three times through depending on your fitness level, then move on to the next sequence.

Sequence #3
- Dumbbell Step-Up on Bench or Step: 10 to 20 reps
- Machine Triceps Push-Down with Rope: 10 to 20 reps
- Incline Reverse Crunch: 10 to 20 reps
- Dip: 10 to 20 reps
- Machine Lower-Back Extension: 10 to 20 reps

Stretch all muscle groups and hold each stretch for at least 30 seconds.

If you're still hungry, run through this "debug" checklist and make sure you're doing everything right.

☐ I am eating all my meals and snacks.

☐ I am measuring my food to ensure the portions are correct.

☐ I am drinking at least 64 ounces of water a day.

☐ I am eating just the food on the list and not adding in other foods.

☐ I am getting at least seven hours of solid sleep per night.

☐ I am exercising for all the designated number of days.

If you did not check all of these, the next day do everything on the list and see if you are still hungry. If you are, consider adding either another snack or a recommended supplement to help curb your appetite. Refer to chapter 5 for more detailed information on what the supplements do and when to take them.

Feeling like you've been doing a good job and need a reward? Or just craving some of your old bad choices? Here's a list of things you can choose from while sticking to your plan (choose only one per day):

Adjust the Exercise Equation

Make it easier. If you feel the exercise is too hard on you, simply cut back the amount of time or the number of days you are doing or reduce the intensity. If you are doing 30 minutes of walking, cut back to 20 minutes, or any amount that makes you feel better. If your resistance training is too difficult, reduce either the amount of weight/resistance you are using, the number of reps you are doing, and/or the number of sets until you feel comfortable. Then continue to progress again at a comfortable pace. If you are a beginner, start with a beginner program, not with the more advanced ones. It will not help you to jump ahead. Be sure to write down the details of your daily workouts so you can track your progress. If you must cut back or reduce your exercise, you must also cut out any reward foods.

Make it harder. If you are a beginner but find the beginner programs to be too easy, first try the progressions, then go ahead and move up to an intermediate program. As long as you can complete the workout safely, with good form and feeling good at the end, you're golden. If you're an intermediate, try some advanced exercises. Check out the box about PHA training on page 135.

- [ ] Up to 5 ounces low-carb frozen yogurt (like Carbowhey or Skinnie Minnie) or another low-carb non-dairy dessert.
- [ ] Up to 2 snack cups (92 grams each) of sugar-free fruit-flavored Jell-O with 1 tablespoon Lite Cool Whip
- [ ] Sugar-free Popsicle
- [ ] Up to 2 sugar-free hot chocolate drinks
- [ ] 1 cup crunchy vegetables (celery, cucumber, radishes, etc.)

What's Next?

Now that you know what to eat, how much to eat, and when to eat, follow the eating plan perfectly. When you lose 20 pounds you will need to recalculate your adjusted total calories. Your ATC will change as you lose weight. Then you will have a whole new set of numbers for your meals (calories, protein, carbs, fat). But again, do not let your calories go below 1,200 per day.

Remember, if you follow the exercise plans, your basal metabolic rate will stay high and you'll lose easier and more consistently. And you will *look* a whole lot better than if you didn't exercise! At the end of the three months you should be at your realistic goal. If you decide you need or want to lose more, continue this plan until you plateau (assuming you are exercising regularly, too). Then, if necessary, move on to one of the stricter, shorter deadline plans. This will bring you quickly to your ultimate goal. Then move on to chapter 10 for maintenance.

7

> > > >

Two Months and Counting

Success means having the courage, the determination, and the will to become the person you believe you were meant to be.

—George Sheehan

By the Numbers

---

2 MONTHS
= 8 WEEKS
= 56 DAYS

How much can you expect to lose?

Pounds: Between 8 and 15

Body fat: 1 to 3 percent

Inches from your waist: 1 to 2

Two months is not a great deal of time, but plenty to make significant changes in your look. Lots of people come to me with only a couple of weeks to make changes in their bodies. Your main focus during these fifty-six days is to make specific adjustments in the way you eat and exercise as well as *the timing of certain meals.* The word *deprived* isn't in my vocabulary, so it shouldn't be in yours, either. However, you will need to be very consistent on this plan. If you had more time, we'd focus on making gradual changes to avoid slipping back into old habits. But with only two months, we need to fine-tune the techniques for slightly faster results.

Although this plan is not as strict as the four- or two-week plans, following it does require discipline and consistency. See how the C word keeps popping up? You will be able to have a variety of foods, as long as you eat them in the required amounts and avoid overindulging. By making good food choices and sticking to the exercise plan that corresponds to your fitness level, you will meet this deadline right on time.

the **EATING** Game Plan at a Glance	Step 1 Pull out your adjusted total calories, which you calculated in chapter 5.
	Step 2 Using the caloric worksheet on pages 141–142, create a framework for your meals that will outline the makeup of your meals—how many calories you will consume in each meal and the protein, fat, nonstarchy vegetable, and complex carbohydrate breakdowns of each.
	Step 3 Pull it all together: look over the food lists and plug in protein, fat, nonstarchy vegetable, and complex carb choices.

Your Custom Eating Plan

Now it's time to plan your meals, one by one, then stick to the plan. You will eat four meals a day, splitting one of the meals in two. One half is to be eaten 40 minutes to 1 hour before your workout and the second half within 30 minutes after your workout. So simply make the meal and divide it in two.

Why eat right before and right after the workout? The pre-workout meal fuels the exercise you are about to do. Too often I see people who are trying to lose weight fall flat on their face during the first half of their workout. It's not the reduced calories that make them run out of gas; it's the timing of the calories they *do* have that makes all the difference. Eat first and you will be able to train longer and harder. The post-workout meal replaces what you've used up. For about an hour after your workout, there's a window of opportunity when your muscles are literally starving for nutrients. The meal you eat at this time is the most important for building muscle and replenishing glycogen (sugar stores in the muscle tissue), which becomes available to you on your next workout.

Remember that skipping meals will not get you there faster, so don't even think about it. In fact, it would be the worst thing you could do. You've got to feed the machine to keep your metabolism stable and to keep those glycogen stores full and ready for the next workout.

To complete the caloric worksheet below, you should know your adjusted total calories—how many calories you can consume and still lose weight. (Refer to chapter 5.) Now you can calculate how many calories should make up each meal. You will further break down the calories in each meal by protein, fat, nonstarchy veggies, and complex carbs. Remember, grams of carbs refers to a combination of veggies and complex carbs.

Caloric Worksheet: Four meals a day _____

_____ ATC ÷ 4 = _____ calories/meal

CARBS PER MEAL

_____ calories/meal × 45% = _____ carbohydrate calories/meal

_____ carbohydrate calories/meal ÷ 4* = _____ carbohydrate grams/meal

There are 4 calories per gram of carbs.

PROTEIN PER MEAL

_____ calories/meal × 35% = _____ protein calories/meal

_____ protein calories/meal ÷ 4* = _____ protein grams/meal

There are 4 calories per gram of protein.

FAT PER MEAL

_____ calories/meal × 20% = _____ fat calories/meal

_____ fat calories/meal ÷ 9* = _____ fat grams/meal

There are 9 calories per gram of fat.

Grams of carbs   = _____ /meal

Grams of protein = _____ /meal

Grams of fat   = _____ /meal

To build your meals, use the list on pages 71–73, to combine (per meal):

One lean protein item

One healthy fat item

One nonstarchy vegetable item

One complex carb item

>>> John's Story

I had been an avid golfer until my back went out. Then I was a mess. My spine was shaped like the letter *S*. I was so bent over that I looked as if I was walking in a windstorm. It was pathetic. And worse, in a matter of weeks, my weight ballooned up to 205 pounds.

I was frustrated with the weight, but also afraid to try anything that might further injure me. One day I was sitting on the couch, probably feeling sorry for myself, watching my wife work out with Gina. Gina looked over at me and asked, "Why don't you join us?"

Because of the back situation, we started out very easy, with just two or three days a week of a lot of stretching, working out gently on an exercise ball to support my back, and a little walking. It was all very controlled. I felt like I was a five-year-old learning everything all over again. But little by little my back started to straighten out. As I got stronger, we increased the intensity of the various exercises, and I could do certain things without a ball. It was all in baby steps, but it worked.

> 66 After a couple of months, I had lost about 25 pounds. But for me, the most important thing was that I had strengthened my back, leg, and stomach muscles and I was no longer in pain. 77
> —JOHN

I also changed my eating. Before, I ate everything, and mainly in restaurants. Because I'm a comedian and either out in the evening or on the road, having a meal once a week at home is a lot for me. And I had two other bad habits: a pack of cigarettes and two candy bars a day—that was my weakness. Gina helped me be more consistent. I learned to eat regular meals throughout the day, cut down on the amount of calories, and add more protein and vegetables. I still snuck candy, but I was mostly sticking to the plan.

After a couple of months, I had lost about 25 pounds. But for me, the most important thing was that I had strengthened my back, leg, and stomach muscles and I was no longer in pain. With Gina, I learned that small steps add up. <<<

Your Custom Exercise Program

Now that you've got your food formula, it's time to put your exercise program into place. Choose the cardio and resistance exercise programs that best suit your current level of fitness.

the EXERCISE Game Plan at a Glance	
Step 1	Determine your exercise level—beginner, intermediate, or advanced. Refer to chapter 3 ("What Kind of Shape Are You In?") to figure out your current fitness level.
Step 2	Look over the workout schedule. You'll do both cardio and resistance training several times a week. You can exercise with equipment or without. If you choose to use equipment, make sure you've got everything you need. I also offer suggestions on how to incorporate exercise machines if that's what you like.
Step 3	Study the illustrations and descriptions of the resistance exercises. This will help you do the workouts properly.
Step 4	Put it all together: be sure to do the proper progression by starting with weeks 1 through 4 at your appropriate exercise level. If you aren't ready to progress, it's also okay to stay on weeks 1 through 4 rather than progressing to weeks 5 through 8.

Important Note: Always check with your physician before starting a new exercise program, especially if you have any medical conditions.

Beginner Workouts

If you're a beginner, you will do this exercise program for eight weeks, including the progressions. Once you can do those, you can then move on to the intermediate programs.

Cardio

BEGINNER: WEEKS 1 THROUGH 8

- Warm up for 5 minutes at 55 percent HR max.
- For weeks 1 through 4, do 20 to 30 minutes at 55 to 75 percent HR max. For weeks 5 through 8 do intervals of 30 seconds at 80

Fit Tips for Beginners

You won't be a beginner for long. The beginner programs will give you a good base of strength and muscle stimulus necessary for the upcoming programs. Follow these suggestions for a better workout:

- Work out at the gym or at home with or without equipment, and stick to the plan. Move on only when it is comfortable for you or you feel you are not getting any more results from the workout you are doing.
- Take the time to look at the pictures and read the exercise descriptions to ensure proper form.
- Always warm up for at least 5 minutes prior to weight training. For best results, stretch at the end of your session.
- Start with a weight that allows you to handle 8 to 12 repetitions with good form.
- Follow the weekly progressions (one set of each exercise the first four weeks, etc.).

- Take the rest periods of 1 to 2 minutes between sets and exercises.
- Perform each exercise in a smooth manner and through a full range of motion.
- Perform each exercise in the sequence it is written. Large muscle groups (such as the legs) are trained first because they require more energy, followed by smaller muscle groups (such as the arms).
- The no equipment workouts can be very strenuous! Don't do them every day. Do your cardio on the alternating days instead.
- Don't be tempted to weight train on consecutive days. Keep a day in between for rest and recovery.
- Do cardio on alternating days as a general rule. If you have to do it on the same day as weight training, do it after your weight workout.

to 85 percent HR max, followed by 3 minutes of active recovery at 55 to 75 percent HR max; repeat for 20 to 30 minutes.

- Cool down for 5 minutes.
- Do cardio six times per week, for 20 minutes after weight training or for 30 minutes on alternating days of weight training.

Weight Training

BEGINNER: WEEKS 1 THROUGH 4

- Warm up with 5 to 10 minutes of continuous cardio exercise, such as walking or stair-climbing.
- Do two sets of 8 to 12 repetitions per exercise.
- Allow 1 to 2 minutes of rest between sets.
- Train on three nonconsecutive days per week: Monday, Wednesday, Friday or Tuesday, Thursday, Saturday.

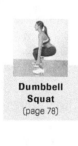

Dumbbell Squat
(page 78)

Stability Ball Leg Curl
(page 79)

Dumbbell Bench Press
(page 79)

Dumbbell One-Arm Row
(page 80)

Dumbbell Biceps Curl
(page 81)

Dumbbell Triceps Kickback
(page 81)

Abdominal Crunch
(page 82)

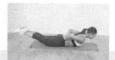

Prone Back Extension with Hands on Lower Back (page 82)

BEGINNER: WEEKS 5 THROUGH 8

- Warm up with 5 to 10 minutes of continuous cardio exercise, such as walking or stair-climbing.
- Do two sets of 8 to 12 repetitions per exercise.

- Allow 1 to 2 minutes of rest between sets.
- Train on three nonconsecutive days per week: Monday, Wednesday, Friday or Tuesday, Thursday, Saturday.

Dumbbell Wall Squat with Stability Ball
(page 83)

Dumbbell Step-Up on Bench or Step
(page 84)

Stability Ball Leg Curl
(page 79)

Dumbbell Bench Press
(page 79)

Dumbbell One-Arm Row
(page 80)

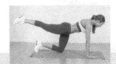

Dumbbell Lateral Raise
(page 85)

Dumbbell Biceps Curl
(page 81)

Dumbbell Triceps Kickback
(page 81)

Abdominal Crunch
(page 82)

One-Leg Hip Extension on All Fours, Alternating
(page 86)

Workout with No Equipment

BEGINNER: WEEKS 1 THROUGH 4

- Warm up with 5 to 10 minutes of continuous cardio exercise, such as walking or stair-climbing.
- Do one set of 10 to 15 repetitions per exercise
- Allow 1 to 2 minutes of rest between sets.
- Train on three nonconsecutive days per week: Monday, Wednesday, Friday or Tuesday, Thursday, Saturday.

Squat with Arms at Sides
(page 93)

Wall Push-Up
(page 93)

Stationary Lunge
(page 94)

Abdominal Crunch
(page 82)

Figure Four
(page 91)

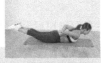

Prone Back Extension with Hands on Lower Back (page 82)

BEGINNER: WEEKS 5 THROUGH 8

- Warm up with 5 to 10 minutes of continuous cardio exercise, such as walking or stair-climbing.
- Do one to two sets of 10 to 15 repetitions per exercise.
- Allow 1 to 2 minutes of rest between sets.
- Train on three nonconsecutive days per week: Monday, Wednesday, Friday or Tuesday, Thursday, Saturday.

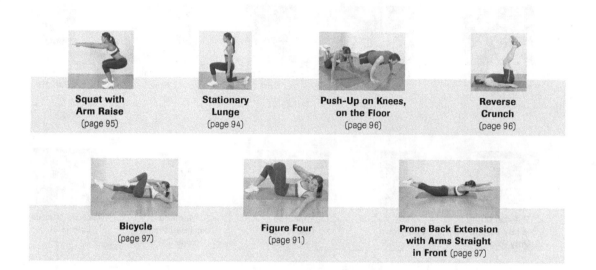

Squat with Arm Raise (page 95)

Stationary Lunge (page 94)

Push-Up on Knees, on the Floor (page 96)

Reverse Crunch (page 96)

Bicycle (page 97)

Figure Four (page 91)

Prone Back Extension with Arms Straight in Front (page 97)

Machine Workouts

If you prefer to work out on machines either at home or the gym, the following lower-body and upper-body machine exercises can be substituted for any of the lower-body/upper-body free-weight exercises mentioned in the preceding pages. Both machines and free weights have their place in a sound exercise program, so use what's most convenient and comfortable for you. As a reminder, go back to chapter 3, reread the advantages and disadvantages of both, and decide what is best for you at this point in time.

Always warm up for 5 to 10 minutes by doing continuous cardio exercise such as walking or stair-climbing before weight training. Perform each exercise with good form, and stretch *after* your workout. Remember, when you use machines, select the weight (or load) that will allow you to perform the exercise in good form for the designated number of repetitions.

Leg Press
(page 98)

Leg Extension
(page 99)

Seated Leg Curl
(page 100)

Seated Cable Row
(page 100)

Assisted Pull-Up
(page 101)

Pull-Up Using Body Weight Only (page 101)

Lat Pull-Down
(page 102)

Machine Chest Fly
(page 102)

Machine Overhead Press
(page 103)

Machine Triceps Extension
(page 104)

Machine Triceps Push-Down with Rope (page 104)

Dip
(page 105)

Machine Biceps Curl
(page 105)

Machine Lower-Back Extension
(page 106)

Machine Abdominal Crunch
(page 106)

Incline Reverse Crunch
(page 107)

Decline Twisting Crunch with Medicine Ball (page 107)

Seated Calf Raise
(page 108)

Make It Harder

Beginners, intermediates, and advanced exercisers: Want to make your current workout more challenging? Add in cardio intervals of 1 to 3 minutes between 8 to 12 repetitions of various exercises and move quickly to and from each one in a circuit-type fashion. This will feel more challenging, increase your heart rate, make your workout more fun and time efficient, and burn more overall calories!

Example:

Warm up by walking on the treadmill for 5 minutes

Dumbbell Squat

Treadmill walking, 2 minutes at a moderate pace

Stability Ball Leg Curl

Treadmill walking, 2 minutes at a moderate pace

Dumbbell Bench Press

Treadmill walking, 2 minutes at a moderate pace

Dumbbell One-Arm Row

Treadmill walking, 2 minutes at a moderate pace

Dumbbell Biceps Curl

Stair-climbing machine, 2 minutes at a moderate pace

Dumbbell Triceps Kickback

Stair-climbing machine, 2 minutes at a moderate pace

Abdominal Crunch

Stair-climbing machine, 2 minutes at a moderate pace

Prone Back Extension with Hands on Lower Back

Stretch

Intermediate Workouts

If you consider yourself an intermediate exerciser, you will follow this workout for eight weeks, including the progressive variations. If you need more of a challenge, you can add advanced exercises from the list beginning on page 153.

Cardio

INTERMEDIATE WEEKS 1 THROUGH 8

- Warm up for 5 minutes at 55 to 75 percent HR max.
- Do intervals. For weeks 1 through 4, do 1 minute at 80 to 85 percent HR max followed by 2 minutes of active recovery at 55

to 75 percent HR max; repeat for 20 to 30 minutes. For weeks 5 through 8, do 2 minutes at 80 to 85 percent HR max, then follow through the sequence as in weeks 1 through 4.

- Do cardio five times per week, for 20 minutes after weight training or for 30 minutes on alternating days of weight training.
- Total workout time, including warm-up and cooldown: 30 minutes on weight-training days, 40 minutes on nonweight-training days.

Fit Tips for Intermediates

Follow these suggestions for a better workout:

- At this stage you can vary the environment in which you do your exercises to stave off boredom.
- Because your goal is fat loss and general fitness, the set and rep scheme is geared toward that. If at any time you change your goal to, say, build strength or put on more muscle, the set and rep scheme would change. For example, lower reps (6 to 8) and heavier loads to build strength, increased volume (more sets) to add bulk.
- Take the time to look at the pictures and read the exercise descriptions to ensure proper technique.
- Always warm up for at least 5 minutes prior to weight training. For best results, stretch at the end of your session.
- Choose weights that allow you to handle the designated number of repetitions with good form.
- Follow the weekly progressions as outlined in the intermediate workout lists.
- Take the rest periods of 2 to 3 minutes between sets and exercises. The harder you train, the longer rest periods you may need, so don't be afraid to rest for up to 4 minutes between sets if you need to.
- Perform each exercise in a smooth manner and through a full range of motion.
- Take note that in this phase of training, the order of some of the exercises is different than in the beginner programs. This is done to give certain muscles a chance to rest before hitting them again in the same workout.
- The no equipment workouts can be very strenuous! Don't do them every day. Do your cardio on alternating days instead.

Weight Training

INTERMEDIATE: WEEKS 1 THROUGH 4

- Warm up with 5 to 10 minutes of continuous cardio exercise, such as walking or stair-climbing.
- Do three sets of 8 to 10 repetitions per exercise.
- Allow 2 to 3 minutes of rest between sets.
- Train on three nonconsecutive days per week: Monday, Wednesday, Friday or Tuesday, Thursday, Saturday.

Dumbbell Squat (page 78)

Dumbbell Bench Press (page 79)

Dumbbell Pull-Over on Stability Ball (page 111)

Overhead Shoulder Press (page 89)

Stability Ball Leg Curl (page 79)

Dumbbell Biceps Curl (page 81)

Lying Dumbbell Triceps Extension (page 90)

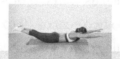

Prone Back Extension with Arms Straight in Front (page 97)

Abdominal Crunch on Stability Ball (page 112)

INTERMEDIATE: WEEKS 5 THROUGH 8

- Warm up with 5 to 10 minutes of continuous cardio exercise, such as walking or stair-climbing.
- Do three sets 8 to 10 repetitions per exercise.
- Allow 2 to 3 minutes of rest between sets.
- Train on three nonconsecutive days per week: Monday, Wednesday, Friday or Tuesday, Thursday, Saturday.

**Dumbbell
Squat Jump**
(page 112)

**Dumbbell Chest
Fly on Ball**
(page 88)

**Dumbbell
One-Arm Row**
(page 80)

**Dumbbell
Lateral Raise**
(page 85)

**Good
Morning**
(page 113)

**Dumbbell Single-Arm
Biceps Curl, Alternating
Arms** (page 90)

**Seated One-Arm
Overhead Triceps
Extension** (page 114)

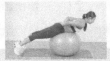

**Back Extension
on Stability Ball**
(page 114)

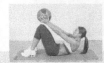

**Weighted Abdominal
Crunch and Reach**
(page 115)

Workout with No Equipment

INTERMEDIATE: WEEKS 1 THROUGH 4

- Warm up with 5 to 10 minutes of continuous cardio exercise, such as walking or stair-climbing.
- Do two sets of 10 to 12 repetitions per exercise.
- Allow 2 to 3 minutes of rest between sets.
- Train on three nonconsecutive days per week: Monday, Wednesday, Friday or Tuesday, Thursday, Saturday.

**Squat with
Arm Raise**
(page 95)

**Push-Up with
T Roll**
(page 116)

**Mountain
Climber**
(page 120)

Pike Press
(page 121)

**One-Leg
Squat Jump**
(page 121)

**Bench/Chair
Triceps Dip**
(page 122)

Bicycle
(page 97)

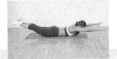

**Prone Back Extension
with Arms Straight
in Front** (page 97)

Lying Side Crunch
(page 123)

INTERMEDIATE: WEEKS 5 THROUGH 8

- Warm up with 5 to 10 minutes of continuous cardio exercise, such as walking or stair-climbing.
- Allow 2 to 3 minutes of rest between sets.
- Do three sets 12 repetitions per exercise.
- Train on three nonconsecutive days per week: Monday, Wednesday, Friday or Tuesday, Thursday, Saturday.

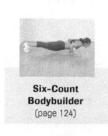

Six-Count Bodybuilder (page 124)

Push-Up with T Roll (page 116)

Mountain Climber (page 120)

Pike Press (page 121)

Stationary Lunge (page 94)

Bench/Chair Triceps Dip with Legs Elevated (page 125)

Crunch with Toe Reach, Legs at 45 Degrees (page 126)

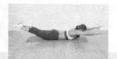

Prone Back Extension with Arms Straight in Front (page 97)

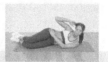

Lying Side Crunch (page 123)

Take It Up a Notch: For Advanced Exercisers

If you're able to perform the intermediate exercises with good form for the designated number of repetitions and sets, and/or you need a cardio boost, follow the instructions in this section for more challenging workouts.

Cardio

ADVANCED: WEEKS 1 THROUGH 8

- Warm up for 5 minutes.
- Do intervals. For weeks 1 through 4, do 3 minutes at 80 to 90 percent HR max followed by 2 minutes of active recovery at 60

to 75 percent HR max; repeat for 20 to 40 minutes. For weeks 5 through 8, do 4 minutes at 80 to 90 percent HR max, then follow through the sequence as in weeks 1 through 4.

- Cool down for 5 minutes.

Take It Up One More Notch with Peripheral Heart Action (PHA) Training

Peripheral Heart Action Training is a variation of circuit training designed to work your cardiovascular system by alternating lower-body exercises with upper-body exercises. This forces the heart to work harder by having to shunt blood up and down the body to the working muscles. It differs from traditional circuit training because you will use moderate to heavy weights instead of lighter weights during a circuit. It can also be done with body weight only to create an amazing cardiovascular and strength workout. The benefits? You'll maximize fat burning and increase postexercise oxygen consumption. You will also get maximum cardiovascular and muscular endurance by keeping blood moving from one body part to the next, not allowing it to pool in any one place for a period of time. Here's how you do it: Take your current workout and order the exercises so that you have a leg or ab/lower-back exercise followed by an upper-body exercise. Repeat this technique with three sequences of four to six exercises. Do between 8 and 20 repetitions with no rest between exercises. You can rest for up to 3 minutes between sequences. The workout would look like this:

Sequence #1
- Dumbbell Squat: 10 to 20 reps
- Abdominal Crunch: 10 to 20 reps
- Push-Up: 10 to 20 reps

- Prone Back Extension with Arms Straight in Front: 10 to 20 reps
- Figure Four: 10 to 20 reps
- Dumbbell Pull-Over on Stability Ball: 10 to 20 reps

Perform the routine one to three times through depending on your fitness level, then move on to the next sequence.

Sequence #2
- Dumbbell Squat Jump: 10 to 20 reps
- Pike Press: 10 to 20 reps
- Leg Press: 10 to 20 reps
- Push-Up with T Roll: 10 to 20 reps
- Machine Abdominal Crunch: 10 to 20 reps

Perform the routine one to three times through depending on your fitness level, then move on to the next sequence.

Sequence #3
- Dumbbell Step-Up on Bench or Step: 10 to 20 reps
- Machine Triceps Push-Down with Rope: 10 to 20 reps
- Incline Reverse Crunch: 10 to 20 reps
- Dip: 10 to 20 reps
- Machine Lower-Back Extension: 10 to 20 reps

Stretch all muscle groups and hold each stretch for at least 30 seconds.

- Do cardio five times per week, for 20 minutes immediately following weight training or for 40 minutes on alternating days.
- Total workout time, including warm-up and cooldown: 30 minutes on weight-training days, 50 minutes on non-weight-training days.

Weight Training

In addition to the exercises you have already learned in the beginner and intermediate programs, you can add or substitute the following exercises to take yourself to a new level of fitness.

- Do three sets of 10 to 12 repetitions per exercise.
- Allow 2 to 3 minutes of rest between sets.
- Train on three nonconsecutive days per week: Monday, Wednesday, Friday or Tuesday, Thursday, Saturday.

Split Jump
(page 128)

Elevated Leg Plank, Alternating Legs (page 128)

Lateral Box Jump-Over (page 129)

Flutter Kick (page 130)

One-Leg Squat Jump (page 121)

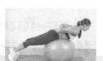
Back Extension on Stability Ball (page 114)

One-Leg Stability Ball Leg Curl (page 130)

Atomic Sit-Up (page 131)

Incline Reverse Crunch (page 107)

Pull-Up using Body Weight Only (page 101)

Decline Twisting Crunch with Medicine Ball (page 107)

Diamond Push-Up (page 132)

Jackknife on Stability Ball (page 132)

Plank (page 122)

Stability Ball Push-Up on Toes (page 133)

Lateral Foam Roll Jump-Over (page 134)

Adjust the Exercise Equation

Make it easier. If you feel the exercise is too hard on you, simply cut back the amount of time or the number of days you are doing or reduce the intensity. If you are doing 30 minutes of walking, cut back to 20 minutes, or any amount that makes you feel better. If your resistance training is too difficult, reduce either the amount of weight/resistance you are using, the number of reps you are doing, and/or the number of sets until you feel comfortable. Then continue to progress again at a comfortable pace. If you are a beginner, start with a beginner program, not with the more advanced ones. It will not help you to jump ahead. Be sure to write down the details of your daily workouts so you can track your progress. If you cut back or reduce your exercise, you must also cut out any reward foods.

Make it harder. If you are a beginner but find the beginner programs to be too easy, first try the progressions, then go ahead and move up to an intermediate program. As long as you can complete the workout safely, with good form and feeling good at the end, you're golden. If you're an intermediate, try some advanced exercises. Check out the box about PHA training on page 154.

Fine-Tuning the Food Formula: What to Do If You Want to Lose More

If you are eating all your meals and therefore all your daily calories, that's great. Do not, I repeat, do *not*, eat less. This will not help you lose more weight. Instead, either add exercise or increase the intensity of the exercise you are currently doing. To do this, choose one of the more difficult workouts if you are up to it. Or increase the intensity of your cardio by walking hills instead of flats; increasing the incline on the treadmill, stair-climber, or elliptical machine; or doing an interval program that I have mapped out for you in the cardio section of this book. But be sure to do only what you can handle.

If you're still hungry, run through this "debug" checklist and make sure you're doing everything right.

- ☐ I am eating all my meals and snacks.
- ☐ I am measuring my food to ensure the portions are correct.
- ☐ I am drinking at least 64 ounces of water a day.

☐ I am eating just the food on the list and not adding in other foods.

☐ I am getting at least seven hours of solid sleep per night.

☐ I am exercising for all the designated number of days.

If you did not check all of these, the next day do everything on the list and see if you are still hungry. If you are, consider adding either another snack or a recommended supplement to help curb your appetite. Refer to chapter 5 for more detailed information on what the supplements do and when to take them.

Feeling like you've been doing a good job and need a reward? Or just craving some of your old bad choices? Here's a list of things you can choose from while sticking to your plan (choose only one per day):

☐ Up to 5 ounces low-carb frozen yogurt (like Carbowhey or Skinnie Minnie) or another low-carb non-dairy dessert

☐ Up to 2 snack cups (92 grams each) sugar-free fruit-flavored Jell-O with 1 tablespoon Lite Cool Whip

☐ Sugar-free Popsicle

☐ Up to 2 sugar-free hot chocolate drinks

☐ 1 cup crunchy vegetables (celery, cucumber, radishes, etc.)

What's Next?

Now that you know what to eat, how much to eat, and when to eat, follow this eating plan perfectly until you lose the estimated 8 to 15 pounds, then recalculate your adjusted total calories. Your ATC will change as you lose weight. Then you will have a whole new set of numbers for your meals (calories, protein, carbs, fat). But again, do not let your calories go below 1,200 per day.

Remember, if you follow the exercise plans, your basal metabolic rate will stay high and you'll lose easier and more consistently. And you will *look* a whole lot better than if you didn't exercise! At the end of the two months you should be at your realistic goal. If you decide you need or want to lose more, continue this plan until you plateau (assuming you are exercising regularly, too). Then, if necessary, move on to one of the stricter, shorter deadline plans. This will bring you quickly to your ultimate goal. Then move on to chapter 10 for maintenance.

8

One Month and Counting

You miss 100 percent of the shots you don't take.

—*Wayne Gretzky*

One month is a great goal if you're going on a vacation and want to shed a few pounds beforehand, or if you're attending an event like a wedding or a reunion. It's definitely enough time to make great strides in your look. But more important, you'll learn better habits that will prep you for the longer life plan ahead. Your main focus during these twenty-eight days is to stick to the plan exactly and adhere to the exercise regimen.

You don't have a lot of leeway here. The shorter deadline calls for more discipline on your part. I have had many clients who have exceeded the best of these results and only the occasional client who fell slightly below the low end of the results. Why? Because with only four weeks to go, you're usually very focused and more disciplined than you are either with a longer deadline or with no deadline at all. But you've got to *earn* this one. This is a strict plan with very specific instructions. You will not have a great variety of foods, but your results will be amazing. This deadline will help you change the worst of your eating habits, then move on to a new deadline: life.

>>> Sally's Story

About a year ago, I shot the pilot for *Army Wives* for Lifetime. When it started looking like the show was going to get picked up,

> In Hollywood, eating disorders are rampant. Anyone can starve herself. I wanted to be in optimal shape, but get there in a healthy way.
> —SALLY

I decided that I needed to get leaner. By the world's standards, I was skinny. I'm five feet two, and I weigh about 100 pounds. But for this character, I wanted to lose a little fat and gain more muscle. Roxy is a sassy, sexy bartender from the wrong side of the tracks. She wears low-cut tops, sky-high heels, and short skirts. So I'd be in front of the camera in almost no clothing for the entire series. That was great motivation.

I had a month, including the holidays when there would be a lot of temptation. My goal was to lose fat in a way that was natural for me. In Hollywood, eating disorders are rampant. Anyone can starve herself. I wanted to be in optimal shape, but get there in a healthy way.

I had always been active and a pretty healthy eater, but once I started working with Gina, I realized that some of my habits needed to change. I would skip breakfast and sometimes eat only one meal a day.

During the first two weeks, I never felt hungry, but I was also never completely full. I guess that's what it's supposed to feel like! I drank a lot of water, which really helped. Still, near the end—as my boyfriend could tell you—there was some definite crankiness. I was really craving a big bowl of ice cream. The maintenance plan was significantly easier to deal with. I was allowed many more foods, including low-carb frozen yogurt. What a relief.

As far as exercise, before the plan, I usually did about 45 minutes of cardio four to five times a week. I would run outside or kickbox, hike, or use the elliptical trainer. But while working I cut the exercise to 45 minutes three days a week. During those maintenance weeks, I added weights so I'd look more toned.

After the first two weeks, my body fat was down 1.5 percent, which was crazy. Even after the month was officially over, I continued on the maintenance plan, and dropped another 2 percent over the next two months. The show did get picked up, and the shoots were often long and grueling. But I felt a lot happier and had much more energy than in the old days, thanks to the program. <<<

---

the EATING Game Plan at a Glance

Step 1 Pull out your adjusted total calories that you calculated in chapter 5.

Step 2 Using the caloric worksheet on page 162, calculate three meals per day plus two protein-only snacks. This framework will tell you how many calories you can consume at each meal, broken down by protein, fat, nonstarchy vegetables, and complex carbohydrates.

Step 3 Pull it all together: look over the food lists and choose your protein, fat, vegetable carb, and complex carb choices.

Your Custom Eating Plan

Now it's time to plan your meals, one by one, then stick to the program.

To complete the caloric worksheet on page 162, you should know your adjusted total calories—how many calories you can consume and still lose weight. (Refer to chapter 5 if you missed that step.) Now you can calculate how many calories should make up each meal. You will further break down the calories in each meal by protein, fat, nonstarchy veggies, and complex carbs. Remember, grams of carbs refers to a combination of veggies and complex carbs. You will also eat two protein-only snacks, and don't save them both for late-night grazing.

Caloric Worksheet:
Three meals with two protein-only snacks _____

_____ ATC × 75% = _____ ÷ 3 meals/day = _____ calories/meal

CARBS PER MEAL

_____ calories/meal × 45% = _____ carbohydrate calories/meal

_____ carbohydrate calories/meal ÷ 4* = _____ carbohydrate grams/meal

*There are 4 calories per gram of carbs.

PROTEIN PER MEAL

_____ calories/meal × 35% = _____ protein calories/meal

_____ protein calories/meal ÷ 4* = _____ protein grams/meal

*There are 4 calories per gram of protein.

FAT PER MEAL

_____ calories/meal × 20% = _____ fat calories/meal

_____ fat calories/meal ÷ 9* = _____ fat grams/meal

*There are 9 calories per gram of fat.

SNACKS

_____ ATC × 25% = _____ ÷ 2 snacks/day = _____ calories/snack

Protein

_____ calories/snack ÷ 4* = _____ protein grams/snack ÷ 2 snacks/day

= _____ protein grams/snack

*There are 4 calories per gram of protein.

Meals		Snacks	
Grams of carbs	= _____ /meal	Grams of protein =	_____ /snack
Grams of protein	= _____ /meal		
Grams of fat	= _____ /meal		

To build your meals, use the list on pages 71–73, to combine (per meal):

One lean protein item

One healthy fat item

One nonstarchy vegetable item

One complex carb item

Your Custom Exercise Program

Now that you've got your food formula, it's time to add in your exercise regimen. Choose the cardio and resistance exercise programs that best suit your current level of fitness.

the EXERCISE Game Plan at a Glance	
Step 1	Determine your exercise level—beginner, intermediate, or advanced. Refer to chapter 3 ("What Kind of Shape Are You In?") to figure out your current fitness level.
Step 2	Look over the workout schedule. You'll do both cardio and resistance training several times a week. You can exercise with equipment or without. If you choose to use equipment, make sure you've got everything you need. I also offer suggestions on how to incorporate exercise machines for variety and convenience.
Step 3	Study the illustrations and descriptions of the resistance exercises. This will help you do the workouts properly.
Step 4	Put it all together: be sure to do the proper progression by starting with weeks 1 and 2 at your appropriate exercise level. If you aren't ready to progress, it's also okay to stay on weeks 1 and 2 rather than progress to weeks 3 and 4.

Important Note: Always check with your physician before starting a new exercise program, especially if you have any medical conditions.

Beginner Workouts

If you're a beginner, you will do this exercise program for one month, including the progressions. Once you can do those, you can then move on to the intermediate programs.

Cardio

BEGINNER: WEEK 1

- Warm up for 5 minutes.
- Do 30 minutes at 55 to 75 percent HR max.
- Cool down for 5 minutes.
- Do cardio three times per week, on alternating days of weight training.

BEGINNER: WEEK 2

- Warm up for 5 minutes at 55 to 75 percent HR max.
- Do intervals of 30 seconds at 80 to 85 percent HR max,

Fit Tips for Beginners

You won't be a beginner for long. The beginner programs will give you a good base of strength and muscle stimulus necessary for the upcoming programs. Follow these suggestions for a better workout:

- Work out at the gym or at home with or without equipment, and stick to the plan. Move on only when it's comfortable for you or you feel you are not getting any more results from the workout you are doing.
- Take the time to look at the pictures and read the exercise descriptions to ensure proper technique.
- Always warm up for at least 5 minutes prior to weight training. For best results, stretch at the end of your session.
- Start with a weight that allows you to handle 8 to 12 repetitions with good form.
- Follow the weekly progressions (one set of each exercise the first two weeks, etc.).

- Take the rest periods of 1 to 2 minutes between sets and exercises
- Perform each exercise in a smooth manner and through a full range of motion.
- Perform each exercise in the sequence it is written. Large muscle groups (such as the legs) are trained first because they require more energy, followed by smaller muscle groups (such as the arms).
- Don't be tempted to weight train on consecutive days. Keep a day in between for rest and recovery.
- Do cardio on alternating days as a general rule. If you have to do it on the same day as weight training, do it after your weight workout.
- The no equipment workouts can be very strenuous! Don't do them every day. Do your cardio on alternating days instead.

followed by 3 minutes of active recovery at 55 to 75 percent HR max; repeat for 20 to 30 minutes.

- Cool down for 5 minutes.
- Do cardio three times per week, on alternating days of weight training.

BEGINNER: WEEKS 3 AND 4

- Warm up for 5 minutes at 55 to 75 percent HR max.
- Do intervals of 30 seconds at 80 to 85 percent HR max, followed by 3 minutes of active recovery at 55 to 75 percent HR max; repeat for 20 to 30 minutes.
- Cool down for 5 minutes.
- Do cardio five times per week, for 20 minutes after weight training or for 30 minutes on alternating days of weight training.

Weight Training

BEGINNER: WEEKS 1 THROUGH 4

- Warm up with 5 to 10 minutes of continuous cardio exercise, such as walking or stair-climbing.
- Do one set of 8 to 12 repetitions per exercise.
- Allow 1 to 2 minutes of rest between sets.
- Train on three nonconsecutive days per week: Monday, Wednesday, Friday or Tuesday, Thursday, Saturday.

| Dumbbell Squat (page 78) | Stability Ball Leg Curl (page 79) | Dumbbell Bench Press (page 79) | Dumbbell One-Arm Row (page 80) | Dumbbell Biceps Curl (page 81) |

**Dumbbell Triceps
Kickback**
(page 81)

**Abdominal
Crunch**
(page 82)

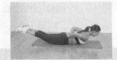

**Prone Back Extension
with Hands on Lower
Back** (page 82)

Workout with No Equipment

BEGINNER: WEEKS 1 THROUGH 4

- Warm up with 5 to 10 minutes of continuous cardio exercise, such as walking or stair-climbing.
- Do one set of 10 to 15 repetitions per exercise.
- Allow 1 to 2 minutes of rest between sets.
- Train on three nonconsecutive days per week: Monday, Wednesday, Friday or Tuesday, Thursday, Saturday.

**Squat with
Arms at Sides**
(page 93)

**Wall
Push-Up**
(page 93)

**Stationary
Lunge**
(page 94)

**Abdominal
Crunch**
(page 82)

Figure Four
(page 91)

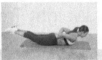

**Prone Back Extension
with Hands on Lower
Back** (page 82)

Machine Workouts

If you prefer to work out on machines either at home or at the gym, the following lower-body and upper-body machine exercises can be substituted for any of the lower-body/upper-body free-weight exercises mentioned in the preceding pages. Both machines and free weights have their place in a sound exercise program, so use what's most convenient and comfortable for you. As a reminder, go back to chapter 3, reread the advantages and disadvantages of both, and decide what is best for you at this point in time.

Always warm up for 5 to 10 minutes by doing continuous cardio exercise such as walking or stair-climbing before weight training. Perform each exercise with good form, and stretch *after* your workout. Remember, when you use machines, select the weight (or load) that allows you to perform the exercise in good form for the designated number of repetitions.

Leg Press
(page 98)

Leg Extension
(page 99)

Seated Leg Curl
(page 100)

Seated Cable Row
(page 100)

Assisted Pull-Up
(page 101)

Lat Pull-Down
(page 102)

Machine Chest Fly
(page 102)

Machine Overhead Press
(page 103)

Machine Triceps Extension
(page 104)

Machine Triceps Push-Down with Rope (page 104)

Dip
(page 105)

Machine Biceps Curl
(page 105)

Machine Lower-Back Extension
(page 106)

Machine Abdominal Crunch
(page 106)

Incline Reverse Crunch
(page 107)

Decline Twisting Crunch with Medicine Ball (page 107)

Seated Calf Raise
(page 108)

Make It Harder

Beginners, intermediates, and advanced exercisers: Want to make your current workout more challenging? Add in cardio intervals of 1 to 3 minutes between 8 to 12 repetition of various exercises and move quickly to and from each one in a circuit-type fashion. This will feel more challenging, increase your heart rate, make your workout more fun and time efficient, and burn more overall calories!

Example:

Warm up by walking on the treadmill for 5 minutes

Dumbbell Squat

Treadmill walking, 2 minutes at a moderate pace

Stability Ball Leg Curl

Treadmill walking, 2 minutes at a moderate pace

Dumbbell Bench Press

Treadmill walking, 2 minutes at a moderate pace

Dumbbell One-Arm Row

Treadmill walking, 2 minutes at a moderate pace

Dumbbell Biceps Curl

Stair-climbing machine, 2 minutes at a moderate pace

Dumbbell Triceps Kickback

Stair-climbing machine, 2 minutes at a moderate pace

Abdominal Crunch

Stair-climbing machine, 2 minutes at a moderate pace

Prone Back Extension with Hands on Lower Back

Stretch

Intermediate Workouts

If you consider yourself an intermediate exerciser, you will follow this workout for four weeks, including the progressive variations. If you need more of a challenge, you can add advanced exercises from the list beginning on page 171.

Cardio

INTERMEDIATE: WEEKS 1 THROUGH 4

- Warm up for 5 minutes at 55 to 75 percent HR max.
- For weeks 1 and 2, do intervals of 1 minute at 80 to 85 percent HR max, followed by 2 minutes of active recovery at

55 to 75 percent HR max; repeat for 20 to 30 minutes. For weeks 3 and 4, do intervals of 2 minutes at 80 to 85 percent HR max, then follow through the sequence as in weeks 1 and 2.

- Cool down for 5 minutes.
- Do cardio five times per week, for 20 minutes after weight training or for 30 minutes on alternating days of weight training. Total workout time, including warm-up and cooldown: 30 minutes on weight-training days, and 40 minutes on non-weight-training days.

Fit Tips for Intermediates

Follow these suggestions for a better workout:

- At this stage you can vary the environment in which you do your exercises to stave off boredom.
- Because your goal is fat loss and general fitness, the set and rep scheme is geared toward that. If at any time you change your goal to, say, build strength or put on more muscle, the set and rep scheme would change. For example, lower reps (6 to 8) and heavier loads to build strength, increased volume (more sets) to add bulk.
- Take the time to look at the pictures and read the exercise descriptions to ensure proper technique.
- Always warm up for at least 5 minutes prior to weight training. For best results, stretch at the end of your weight-training session.
- Choose weights that allow you to handle

the designated number of repetitions with good form.

- Take the rest periods of 2 to 3 minutes between sets and exercises. The harder you train, the longer rest periods you may need, so don't be afraid to rest for up to 4 minutes between sets if you need to.
- Perform each exercise in a smooth manner and through a full range of motion.
- Take note that in this phase of training, the order of some of the exercises is different than in the beginner programs. This is done to give certain muscles a chance to rest before hitting them again in the same workout.
- The no equipment workouts can be very strenuous! Don't be tempted to do them every day. Do your cardio on alternating days instead.

Weight Training

INTERMEDIATE: WEEKS 1 THROUGH 4

- Warm up with 5 to 10 minutes of continuous cardio exercise, such as walking or stair-climbing.
- Do three sets of 8 to 10 repetitions per exercise.
- Allow 1 to 2 minutes of rest between sets.
- Train on three nonconsecutive days per week: Monday, Wednesday, Friday or Tuesday, Thursday, Saturday.

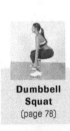

Dumbbell Squat (page 78)

Dumbbell Bench Press (page 79)

Dumbbell Pull-Over on Stability Ball (page 111)

Overhead Shoulder Press (page 89)

Stability Ball Leg Curl (page 79)

Dumbbell Biceps Curl (page 81)

Lying Dumbbell Triceps Extension (page 90)

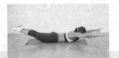

Prone Back Extension with Arms Straight in Front (page 97)

Weighted Lateral Crunch on Stability Ball (page 112)

Workout with No Equipment

INTERMEDIATE: WEEKS 1 THROUGH 4

- Warm up for 5 to 10 minutes with continuous cardio exercise, such as walking or stair-climbing.
- Do two sets of 10 to 12 repetitions per exercise.
- Allow 1 to 2 minutes of rest between sets.
- Train on three nonconsecutive days per week: Monday, Wednesday, Friday or Tuesday, Thursday, Saturday.

Stationary Lunge
(page 94)

Push-Up with T Roll
(page 116)

Mountain Climber
(page 120)

Pike Press
(page 121)

One-Leg Squat Jump
(page 121)

Bench/Chair Triceps Dip
(page 122)

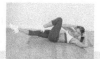

Bicycle
(page 97)

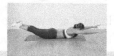

Prone Back Extension with Arms Straight in Front (page 97)

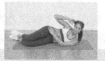

Lying Side Crunch
(page 123)

Take It Up a Notch: For Advanced Exercisers

If you're able to perform the intermediate exercises with good form for the designated number of repetitions and sets, and/or you need a cardio boost, follow the instructions for more challenging workouts in this section:

Cardio

ADVANCED: WEEKS 1 THROUGH 4

- Warm up for 5 minutes.
- Do intervals. For weeks 1 and 2, do 3 minutes at 80 to 90 percent HR max, followed by 2 minutes of active recovery at 60 to 75 percent HR max; repeat for 20 to 40 minutes. For weeks 3 and 4, do 4 minutes at 80 to 90 percent HR max, then follow through the sequence as in weeks 1 and 2.
- Cool down for 5 minutes.
- Do cardio five times per week, for 20 minutes immediately following weight training or for 40 minutes on alternating days.

- Total workout time, including warm-up and cooldown: 30 minutes on weight-training days, 50 minutes on non-weight-training days.

Take It Up One More Notch with Peripheral Heart Action (PHA) Training

Peripheral Heart Action Training is a variation of circuit training designed to work your cardiovascular system by alternating lower-body exercises with upper-body exercises. This forces the heart to work harder by having to shunt blood up and down the body to the working muscles. It differs from traditional circuit training because you will use moderate to heavy weights instead of lighter weights during a circuit. It can also be done with body weight only to create an amazing cardiovascular and strength workout. The benefits? You'll maximize fat burning and increase postexercise oxygen consumption. You will also get maximum cardiovascular and muscular endurance by keeping blood moving from one body part to the next, not allowing it to pool in any one place for a period of time. Here's how you do it: Take your current workout and order the exercises so that you have a leg or ab/lower-back exercise followed by an upper-body exercise. Repeat this technique with three sequences of four to six exercises. Do between 8 and 20 repetitions with no rest between exercises. You can rest for up to 3 minutes between sequences. The workout would look like this:

Sequence #1

- Dumbbell Squat: 10 to 20 reps
- Abdominal Crunch: 10 to 20 reps
- Push-Up: 10 to 20 reps
- Prone Back Extension with Arms Straight in Front: 10 to 20 reps
- Figure Four: 10 to 20 reps
- Dumbbell Pull-Over on Stability Ball: 10 to 20 reps

Perform the routine one to three times through depending on your fitness level, then move on to the next sequence.

Sequence #2

- Dumbbell Squat Jump: 10 to 20 reps
- Pike Press; 10 to 20 reps
- Leg Press: 10 to 20 reps
- Push-Up with T Roll: 10 to 20 reps
- Machine Abdominal Crunch: 10 to 20 reps

Perform the routine one to three times through depending on your fitness level, then move on to the next sequence.

Sequence #3

- Dumbbell Step-Up on Bench or Step: 10 to 20 reps
- Machine Triceps Push-Down with Rope: 10 to 20 reps
- Incline Reverse Crunch: 10 to 20 reps
- Dip: 10 to 20 reps
- Machine Lower-Back Extension: 10 to 20 reps

Stretch all muscle groups and hold each stretch for at least 30 seconds.

Weight Training

In addition to the exercises you have already learned in the beginner and intermediate programs, you can add or substitute the following exercises to take yourself to a new level of fitness.

- Do three sets of 10 to 12 repetitions per exercise.
- Allow 1 to 2 minutes of rest between sets.
- Train on three nonconsecutive days per week: Monday, Wednesday, Friday or Tuesday, Thursday, Saturday.

Split Jump
(page 128)

Elevated Leg Plank, Alternating Legs (page 128)

Lateral Box Jump-Over
(page 129)

Flutter Kick
(page 130)

One-Leg Squat Jump
(page 121)

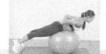
Back Extension on Stability Ball
(page 114)

One-Leg Stability Ball Leg Curl
(page 130)

Atomic Sit-Up
(page 131)

Incline Reverse Crunch
(page 107)

Pull-Up Using Body Weight Only (page 101)

Decline Twisting Crunch with Medicine Ball (page 107)

Diamond Push-Up
(page 132)

Jackknife on Stability Ball
(page 132)

Stability Ball Push-Up, on Toes
(page 133)

Lateral Foam Roll Jump-Over (page 134)

Adjust the Exercise Equation

Make it easier. If you feel the exercise is too hard on you, simply cut back the amount of time or the number of days you are doing or reduce the intensity. If you are doing 30 minutes of walking, cut back to 20 minutes, or any amount that makes you feel better. If your resistance training is too difficult, reduce either the amount of weight/resistance you are using, the number of reps you are doing, and/or the number of sets until you feel comfortable. Then continue to progress again at a comfortable pace. If you are a beginner start with a beginner program, not with the more advanced ones. It will not help you to jump ahead. Be sure to write down the details of your daily workouts so you can track your progress. If you cut back or reduce your exercise, you must also cut out any reward foods.

Make it harder. If you are a beginner but find the beginner programs to be too easy, first try the progressions, then go ahead and move up to an intermediate program. As long as you can complete the workout safely, with good form and feeling good at the end, you're golden. If you're an intermediate, try some advanced exercises. Check out the box about PHA training on page 172.

Fine-Tuning the Food Formula: What to Do If You Want to Lose More

If you are eating all your meals and therefore all your daily calories, that's great. Do not, I repeat, do *not*, eat less. This will not help you to lose more weight. Instead, either add exercise or increase the intensity of the exercise you are currently doing. To do this, choose one of the more difficult workouts if you are up to it. Or increase the intensity of your cardio by walking hills instead of flats; increasing the incline on the treadmill, stair-climber, or elliptical machine; or doing an interval program that I have mapped out for you in this chapter. But be sure to do only what you can handle.

If you're still hungry, run through this "debug" checklist and make sure you're doing everything right.

☐ I am eating all my meals and snacks.

☐ I am measuring my food to ensure the portions are correct.

☐ I am drinking at least 64 ounces of water a day.

☐ I am eating just the food on the list and not adding in other foods.

☐ I am getting at least seven hours of solid sleep per night.

☐ I am exercising for all the designated number of days.

If you did not check all of these, the next day do everything on the list and see if you are still hungry. If you are, consider adding either another snack or a recommended supplement to help curb your appetite. Refer to chapter 5 for detailed info on what the supplements do and when to take them.

Feeling like you've been doing a good job and need a reward? Or just craving some of your old bad choices? Here's a list of things you can choose from while sticking to your plan (choose only one per day):

☐ Up to 5 ounces low-carb frozen yogurt (like Carbowhey or Skinnie Minnie) or a low-carb non-dairy dessert

☐ Up to 2 snack cups (92 grams each) sugar-free fruit-flavored Jell-O with 1 tablespoon Lite Cool Whip

☐ Sugar-free Popsicle

☐ Up to 2 sugar-free hot chocolate drinks

☐ 1 cup crunchy vegetables (celery, cucumber, radishes, etc.)

What's Next?

Now that you know what to eat, how much to eat, and when to eat, follow this eating plan perfectly until you lose the estimated 4 to 13 pounds, then recalculate your adjusted total calories. Your ATC will change as you lose weight. Then you will have a whole new set of numbers for your meals (calories, protein, carbs, fat). But again, do not let your calories go below 1,200 per day.

Remember, if you follow the exercise plans, your basal metabolic rate will stay high and you'll lose easier and more consistently. And you will *look* a whole lot better than if you didn't exercise! At the end of the four weeks you should be at your realistic goal. If you decide you need or want to lose more, continue this plan until you plateau (assuming you are exercising regularly, too). Then, if necessary, move on to the two-week plan. This will bring you quickly to your ultimate goal. Then move on to chapter 10 for maintenance.

9

Two Weeks and Counting

It is astonishing how short a time it takes for very wonderful things to happen.

—Frances Burnett

By the Numbers

2 WEEKS
= 14 DAYS

How much can you expect to lose?

Pounds: Between 2 and 8

Body fat: 1 to 1.5 percent

Inches from your waist: ½ to 1

This is probably the plan that people request most often. It's the "You got the job" call followed by "Oh no—how do I lose five or ten pounds in the shortest time possible? And do it safely without starving myself!"

With only two weeks to work with, you *must* be more focused and disciplined than you have ever been before. *This deadline is the strictest of them all and not for the weak-willed.* You will learn how to test yourself. Following this plan requires sacrifice in the way of choices, but the results are tremendous! Needless to say, how much you lose will depend on how hard you work. If you can do this, you can probably do anything.

This plan is also a great choice if you need to lose those last stubborn 5 or 10 pounds. The two weeks may be grueling, but maintenance is something to look forward to. And you *will* look forward to it.

You should *not* follow this plan for more than two weeks. If you have met your goal after these fourteen days, immediately go on to the maintenance plan (in chapter 10) as your lifelong plan. If you need to lose more, choose another plan (say the one-month deadline) to achieve the rest of your results. Then move on to the maintenance plan.

Your main focus during these two weeks is to stick to the plan exactly, with *no* substitutions or alterations. It is strict, with very specific instructions. The key in such a short-term plan is utilizing stored body fat as much as possible. Adhere to the exercise program you have chosen based on your current fitness level. Do not choose a tougher exercise plan thinking it will get you to your goal faster. It won't. It will only get you benched.

This deadline will help you change the worst of your eating habits, then move on to a new deadline: life. Down the road, you can think of this two-week plan as your "jump starter." If you ever derail, you can get on it again and make a fresh start toward good eating and exercise habits. (If you ever need to use this plan again, you should wait at least four to six weeks before restarting.)

⟩⟩⟩ Kathryn's Story

I came to Gina with the goal of becoming firmer and leaner. I was already an avid exerciser, but I wasn't as good in the eating department. I was a notorious breakfast and lunch skipper. I never bought into the whole "eat regularly" rule, even though I read it a million times. That didn't work for me. I find eating in the morning gross, so a lot of times I wasn't eating until afternoon. Then I'd be ravenously hungry and also self-righteous, so I'd eat anything.

I hadn't intended to do it so quickly, but when Gina asked me, "What's your goal?" I told her, "As soon as possible; let's just do it!"

As an actress, I'm really good at crash dieting for a certain event, like the Emmys. Since that was easy, I thought I'd go that route and try the intense "step up, step down" program while also learning a healthy way to stay lean.

> ❝ I hadn't intended to do it so quickly, but when Gina asked me, 'What's your goal?' I told her, 'As soon as possible; let's just do it!' ❞
> —KATHRYN

For the two weeks, some days I'd eat only protein and vegetables, and then some days I'd add in some additional healthy carbs. The biggest change was eating more often. Since I wasn't used to eating in the morning, Gina put me on protein shakes to help me deal with breakfast. They ended up being great, and helped me stabilize my blood sugar.

The first couple of days were really hard, and I had to be very disciplined. I really craved sweets and dry, crunchy foods. But I was encouraged when, right away, I lost weight—three pounds in three days. So I began to feel pretty darn good.

As far as my workouts, I continued taking cardio dance classes five or six days a week and Pilates, but added resistance training. I also did interval workouts on the elliptical trainer and some circuit training. Once the fat started coming off, my legs especially looked great!

After the two weeks, my body had shrunk. Everything was still there, but it was just smaller and tighter. I was losing everywhere. I went shopping for new clothes and suddenly all these styles were flattering. Things were smoother and firmer, and that was very gratifying.

It was interesting; I really didn't lose all that much weight, but in the two weeks, my body fat went from 24 to 18 percent. In another two weeks, on a less strict program, I was down to 14 percent body fat.

Now that I'm off that plan and on maintenance, I'm working on keeping things in balance. I'm eating more often and in a more focused way. I got a digital food scale, so I have a sense of what different portion sizes are. The hardest thing is moderation, but overall I'm very happy with where I'm at. ‹‹‹

Your Custom Eating Plan

For the two weeks, you will follow the Stair-Step Formula. This plan is strict, but always yields the fastest and most dramatic results. Years ago, I used it with bodybuilders. Have you ever seen a fat body-builder? This plan is tremendous if you eat the right amounts of lean protein, vegetables, and complex carbs. Always, always, always eat consistently and drink lots of water.

the EATING Game Plan at a Glance	
Step 1	Depending on your current weight, choose the portion sizes that fit you.
Step 2	Read over the limited list of foods and start planning your meals.
Step 3	Do not eat out during these two weeks if possible.
Step 4	Have the "extras" only if you need them.
	Remember that skipping meals will not get you there faster, so don't even think about it!

If you're wondering what the "stair-step technique" means, you're not alone. Most people have no idea and assume that it means they have to do some crazy stair-climbing workout!

Stair-stepping refers to the amount and kind of carbs you'll eat each day. For the first couple of days you'll "step down" by eating carbs only from vegetable sources. On the "step-up" days, you'll get to eat starchier carbs (other than vegetables) for the first and third meals. This method works by keeping the body fed, but with the cleanest, most complex foods. It is fat-free and also very low in the starchier carbs most of us crave.

A note of caution: Stair-stepping works extremely well, but can only be used temporarily. Since your body needs healthy fats to function properly, you should not stay on this plan more than two weeks. So you have to promise me that. If you want to do the plan more than once, you need to give yourself four to six weeks in between. If you use it more often, your metabolism will slow down and you won't get the same great results the second time. So please don't disregard the warnings not to repeat this program more than twice per year.

After the initial fourteen days, move on to another plan or on to maintenance if you've reached your goal. You will not figure out your basal metabolic rate or adjusted total calories for this plan since it is very short-term. Instead, I calculate the portions of protein, carbs, and vegetable carbs you will be eating. This is the only plan for which you will not have to do the math. We will further break down the calories in each meal to grams of protein, nonstarchy veggies, and complex carbs. (Remember, there is no fat on this two-week plan at all, only carbs and protein.) You'll be feeling it on this plan, but the deadline is short, and you'll be glad you toughed it out for the fourteen days!

Determining Your Portion Sizes for Each Meal

Since women generally have less muscle mass than men, they will require slightly less protein at each meal.

If you are a woman who weighs between 100 and 150 pounds, you will have the following at each meal:

28 protein grams (e.g., 4 ounces of fish, chicken, etc., on step-up and step-down days)

20 carbohydrate grams (e.g., ¼ cup oatmeal at meals 1 and 3 on step-up days only)

10 vegetable carbohydrate grams (e.g., 1 cup broccoli on step-down days and meals 2 and 4 on step-up days)

If you are a woman who weighs between 150 and 200 pounds (or more), you will have the following at each meal:

35 protein grams (e.g., 5 ounces of fish, chicken, etc., on step-up and step-down days)

20 carbohydrate grams (e.g., ¼ cup oatmeal at meals 1 and 3 on step-up days only)

20 vegetable carbohydrate grams (e.g., 1½ cups broccoli on step-down days and at meals 2 and 4 on step-up days)

If you are a man who weighs up to 165 pounds, you will have the following at each meal:

40 protein grams (e.g., 6 ounces of fish, chicken, etc., on step-up and step-down days)

25 carbohydrate grams (e.g., ¾ cup oatmeal at meals 1 and 3 on step-up days only)

20 vegetable carbohydrate grams (e.g., 1½ cups broccoli on step-down days and meals 2 and 4 on step-up days)

If you are a man who weighs more 165 pounds, you will have:

50 protein grams (e.g., 7 ounces of fish, chicken, etc., on step-up and step-down days)

35 carbohydrate grams (e.g., 1 cup oatmeal at meals 1 and 3 on step-up days only)

25 vegetable carbohydrate grams (e.g., 2 cups broccoli on step-down days and at meals 2 and 4 on step-up days)

When planning your meals, refer to pages 183–185 for detailed information on how many grams of protein, carbohydrates, and vegetable carbohydrates are in the foods on the list. The Stair-Step Formula worksheet on this page will help you keep track of when you step up and when you step down. You can use the space after each step-up and step-down day to fill in the corresponding date during your two-week deadline period.

The Stair-Step Formula

1 Step down	_____	8 Step up	_____
2 Step down	_____	9 Step up	_____
3 Step up	_____	10 Step down	_____
4 Step up	_____	11 Step down	_____
5 Step down	_____	12 Step down	_____
6 Step down	_____	13 Step down	_____
7 Step up	_____	14 Step down	_____

How to Put Together the Step-Up and Step-Down Meals

On step-down days, choose one protein item and one vegetable item for each of the four meals. Make sure to prepare your food using as little fat as possible. That means grilled, baked, or broiled with no skin, no oil, and no butter.

Step-Down Day Proteins: one serving per meal

Chicken (7 grams per ounce)

Egg whites, measured raw (3 grams per white)

Fish, any kind (7 grams per ounce)

Lean turkey breast or ground turkey patties (7 grams per ounce)

Shellfish, including shrimp (7 grams per ounce)

Sushi, fish only (no rice), including seaweed wraps (7 grams per ounce)

Tofu, silken or firm (2 grams per ounce—watch the fat content)

Whey protein powder shake or any ion-exchange whey powder that has no carbs or fat, made with water and ice (check the label for protein grams)

Step-Down Day Vegetables: one serving per meal

Asparagus (1 spear = 1 gram)

Bell peppers—red, green, orange (12 grams per whole large pepper)

Broccoli (1 cup = 6 grams)

Cauliflower (1 cup cooked = 5 grams)

Green beans (1 cup = 8 grams)

Mushrooms (1 cup = 2 grams)

Onions (1 cup = 15 grams)

Organic lettuces, any kind (1 cup = 2 grams)

Squash/zucchini/cucumber (1 cup = 4 grams)

Tomatoes (1 medium = 5 grams)

On step-up days, choose one protein item for all four meals and one carbohydrate item for the first and third meals only. You will have one vegetable item at the second and fourth meals.

Step-Up Day Proteins: one serving per meal

Chicken (7 grams per ounce)

Egg whites, measured raw (3 grams per white)

Fish, any kind (7 grams per ounce)

Lean turkey breast or ground turkey patties (7 grams per ounce)

Shellfish, including shrimp (7 grams per ounce)

Sushi, fish only (no rice), including seaweed wrap (7 grams per ounce)

Tofu, silken or firm (2 grams per ounce—watch the fat content)

Whey protein powder shake or any ion-exchange whey powder that has no carbs or fat, made with water and ice (check the label for protein grams)

Step-Up Day Carbohydrates: one serving at first and third meals

Apple (1 cup slices = 25 grams)

Beans/legumes, any kind (1 cup = 38 grams)

Berries (1 cup = 12 grams)

Brown rice, cooked (1 cup = 45 grams)

High-fiber cereal, like Fiber One, with ½ cup nonfat organic milk (½ cup cereal = 25 grams; ½ cup nonfat milk = 7 grams)

Oatmeal, made with water (½ cup = 27 grams)

Red potatoes (1 cup = 37 grams)

Wheat tortilla or wheat lavash (1½ ounces = 23 grams)

Yam/sweet potato (1 cup = 37 grams)

Step-Up Day Vegetables: one serving at second and fourth meals

Asparagus (1 spear = 1 gram)

Bell peppers—red, green, orange (12 grams per whole large pepper)

Broccoli (1 cup = 6 grams)

Cauliflower (1 cup cooked = 5 grams)

Green beans (1 cup = 8 grams)

Mushrooms (1 cup = 2 grams)

Onions (1 cup = 15 grams)

Organic lettuces, any kind (1 cup = 2 grams)

Squash/zucchini/cucumber (1 cup = 4 grams)

Tomatoes (1 medium = 5 grams)

Note: Nutritional data in parentheses was taken from www.nutritiondata.com.

Extras

Eat these only if absolutely necessary!

1 cup strawberries per day or one small apple

1 sugar-free Popsicle (not the no-sugar-added type; they are still loaded with sugar!)

Sliced cucumbers or celery, up to 1 cup

Mixed lettuce salad (up to 2 cups) with vinegar only

Coming Off the Two-Week Deadline Plan

Because this is a very strict plan, your body will need some adjustment time when coming off the eating regimen. It doesn't mean you will gain back all the weight that you just lost, but expect the scale to fluctuate between 1 and 4 pounds on the first few days of the next plan you go on. This is normal. You will begin to lose weight again as you groove into the next phase of eating. Choose your next plan based on what your new goal is. If it's a long-term goal, go with the three-month deadline plan and then move on to maintenance (see chapter 10). If you still have a few more pounds to lose quickly, go to the one-month or two-month deadline plans and then on to maintenance.

Do not go from this two-week plan on to the emergency one-week plan outlined later in this chapter. This would dramatically reduce your long-term results! In fact, it could cause you to *gain* weight. Really. We don't want your body to adjust to the lower intake of calories. Remember, the body needs to be fueled consistently. Very short-term plans are just that . . . short term!

Your Custom Exercise Program

Now that you're clear on what you're eating, it's time to put your exercise program into place. Choose the cardio and resistance exercise programs that best suit your current level of fitness.

---

the EXERCISE Game Plan at a Glance

Step 1 Determine your exercise level—beginner, intermediate, or advanced. Refer to chapter 3 ("What Kind of Shape Are You In?") to figure out your current fitness level.

Step 2 Look over the workout schedule. You'll do both cardio and resistance training several times a week. You can exercise with equipment or without. If you choose to use equipment, make sure you've got everything you need. I also offer suggestions on how to incorporate exercise machines for variety and convenience.

Step 3 Study the illustrations and descriptions of the resistance exercises. This will help you do the workouts properly.

Step 4 Progression is an important part of a solid long-term program that yields results. But on this short deadline there is no room for progression. You will progress your routines when you are either on a longer deadline program or on maintenance.

Important note: Always check with your physician before starting a new exercise program, especially if you have any medical conditions.

Beginner Workouts

If you're a beginner, you will do this exercise program for two weeks. Then you will move on to the exercise plan corresponding to your new deadline, whether it is maintenance or another longer-term deadline plan in this book.

Fit Tips for Beginners

You won't be a beginner for long. The beginner programs will give you a good base of strength and muscle stimulus necessary for the upcoming programs. Follow these suggestions for a better workout:

- Work out at the gym or at home with or without equipment, and stick to the plan. Move on only when it is comfortable for you or you feel you are not getting any more results from the workout you are doing.

- Take the time to look at the pictures and read the exercise descriptions to ensure proper technique.

- Always warm up for at least 5 minutes prior to weight training. For best results, stretch at the end of your session.

- Start with a weight that allows you to handle 8 to 12 repetitions with good form.

- Take the rest periods of 1 to 2 minutes between sets and exercises.

- Perform each exercise in a smooth manner and through a full range of motion.

- Perform each exercise in the sequence it is written. Large muscle groups (such as the legs) are trained first because they require more energy, followed by smaller muscle groups (such as the arms).

- Don't be tempted to weight train on consecutive days. Keep a day in between for rest and recovery.

- Do cardio on alternating days as a general rule. If you have to do it on the same day as weight training, do it after your weight workout.

- The no equipment workouts can be very strenuous! Don't do them every day. Do your cardio on alternating days instead.

Cardio

- Warm up for 5 minutes at 55 to 75 percent HR max.
- Do 15 minutes at 55 to 75 percent HR max, followed by 15 minutes of intervals of 30 seconds at 80 to 85 percent HR max, followed by 2 minutes of active recovery at 55 to 75 percent HR max.
- Cool down for 5 minutes.
- Do cardio three to five times per week depending on your energy level, on opposite days of weight training. On weight-training days, do cardio after weights.

Weight Training

- Warm up with 5 to 10 minutes of continuous cardio exercise, such as walking or stair-climbing.
- Do one set of 8 to 12 repetitions per exercise.
- Train on three nonconsecutive days per week: Monday, Wednesday, Friday or Tuesday, Thursday, Saturday.
- Allow 1 to 2 minutes of rest between sets.

Dumbbell Squat
(page 78)

Stability Ball Leg Curl
(page 79)

Dumbbell Bench Press
(page 79)

Dumbbell One-Arm Row
(page 80)

Dumbbell Biceps Curl
(page 81)

Dumbbell Triceps Kickback
(page 81)

Abdominal Crunch
(page 82)

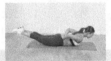

Prone Back Extension with Hands on Lower Back (page 82)

Workout with No Equipment

- Warm up with 5 to 10 minutes of continuous cardio exercise, such as walking or stair-climbing.
- Do one set of 10 to 15 repetitions per exercise.
- Allow 1 to 2 minutes of rest between sets.
- Train on three nonconsecutive days per week: Monday, Wednesday, Friday or Tuesday, Thursday, Saturday.

Squat with Arms at Sides
(page 93)

Wall Push-Up
(page 93)

Stationary Lunge
(page 94)

Abdominal Crunch
(page 82)

Figure Four
(page 91)

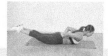
Prone Back Extension with Hands on Lower Back (page 82)

Machine Workouts

If you prefer to work out on machines either at home or at the gym, the following lower-body and upper-body machine exercises can be substituted for any of the lower-body/upper-body free-weight exercises mentioned in the preceding pages. Both machines and free weights have their place in a sound exercise program, so it's best to use what's most convenient and comfortable for you. As a reminder, go back to chapter 3, reread the advantages and disadvantages of both, and decide what is best for you at this point in time.

Always warm up for 5 to 10 minutes by doing continuous cardio exercise like walking or stair-climbing before weight training. Perform each exercise with good form, and stretch *after* your workout. Remember, when you use machines, select the weight (or load) that will allow you to perform the exercise in good form for the designated number of repetitions.

Leg Press
(page 98)

Leg Extension
(page 99)

Seated Leg Curl
(page 100)

Seated Cable Row
(page 100)

Assisted Pull-Up
(page 101)

Pull-Up Using Body Weight Only
(page 101)

Lat Pull-Down
(page 102)

Machine Chest Fly
(page 102)

Machine Overhead Press
(page 103)

Machine Triceps Extension
(page 104)

Machine Triceps Push-Down with Rope (page 104)

Dip (page 105)

Machine Biceps Curl (page 105)

Machine Lower-Back Extension (page 106)

Machine Abdominal Crunch (page 106)

Incline Reverse Crunch (page 107)

Decline Twisting Crunch with Medicine Ball (page 107)

Seated Calf Raise (page 108)

Make It Harder

Beginners, intermediates, and advanced exercisers: Want to make your current workout more challenging? Add in cardio intervals of 1 to 3 minutes between 8 to 12 repetitions of various exercises and move quickly to and from each one in a circuit-type fashion. This will feel more challenging, increase your heart rate, make your workout more fun and time efficient, and burn more overall calories!

Example:

Warm up by walking on the treadmill for 5 minutes

Dumbbell Squat

Treadmill walking, 2 minutes at a moderate pace

Stability Ball Leg Curl

Treadmill walking, 2 minutes at a moderate pace

Dumbbell Bench Press

Treadmill walking, 2 minutes at a moderate pace

Dumbbell One-Arm Row

Treadmill walking, 2 minutes at a moderate pace

Dumbbell Biceps Curl

Stair-climbing machine, 2 minutes at a moderate pace

Dumbbell Triceps Kickback

Stair-climbing machine, 2 minutes at a moderate pace

Abdominal Crunch

Stair-climbing machine, 2 minutes at a moderate pace

Prone Back Extension with Hands on Lower Back

Stretch

Intermediate Workouts

If you consider yourself an intermediate exerciser, you will follow this workout for two weeks, then move on to the exercise program corresponding to your new deadline—whether it is maintenance or another longer-term deadline plan. If you need more of a challenge, you can add advanced exercises from the list beginning on page 193.

Fit Tips for Intermediates

Follow these suggestions for a better workout:

- At this stage you can vary the environment in which you do your exercises to stave off boredom.

- Because your goal is fat loss and general fitness, the set and rep scheme is geared toward that. If at any time you change your goal to, say, build strength or put on more muscle, the set and rep scheme would change. For example, lower reps (6 to 8) and heavier loads to build strength, increased volume (more sets) to add bulk.

- Take the time to look at the pictures and read the exercise descriptions to ensure proper technique.

- Always warm up for at least 5 minutes prior to weight training. For best results, stretch at the end of your weight-training session.

- Choose weights that allow you to handle the designated number of repetitions with good form.

- Take the rest periods of 2 to 3 minutes between sets and exercises. The harder you train, the longer rest periods you may need, so don't be afraid to rest for up to 4 minutes between sets if you need to.

- Perform each exercise in a smooth manner and through a full range of motion.

- Take note that in this phase of training, the order of some of the exercises is different than in the beginner programs. This is done to give certain muscles a chance to rest before hitting them again in the same workout.

- The no equipment workouts can be very strenuous! Don't be tempted to do them every day. Do your cardio on alternating days instead.

Cardio

- Warm up for 5 minutes at 55 to 75 percent HR max.
- Do 40 minutes of intervals: 3 minutes at 80 to 90 percent HR max, followed by 2 minutes of active recovery at 60 to 75 percent HR max, repeated 8 times.

- Cool down for 5 minutes.
- Do cardio five times per week, after weight training on weight-training days. Total workout time, including warm-up and cooldown: 50 minutes.

Weight Training

- Warm up with 5 to 10 minutes of continuous cardio exercise, such as walking or stair-climbing.
- Do three sets of 8 to 10 repetitions per exercise.
- Allow 1 to 2 minutes of rest between sets.
- Train on three nonconsecutive days per week: Monday, Wednesday, Friday or Tuesday, Thursday, Saturday.

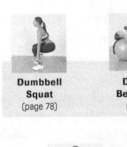

Dumbbell Squat (page 78)

Dumbbell Bench Press (page 79)

Dumbbell Pull-Over on Stability Ball (page 111)

Overhead Shoulder Press (page 89)

Stability Ball Leg Curl (page 79)

Dumbbell Biceps Curl (page 81)

Lying Dumbbell Triceps Extension (page 90)

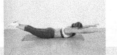

Prone Back Extension with Arms Straight in Front (page 97)

Weighted Lateral Crunch on Stability Ball (page 119)

Workout with No Equipment

- Warm up with 5 to 10 minutes of continuous cardio exercise, such as walking or stair-climbing.
- Do two sets of 10 to 12 repetitions per exercise.

- Allow 1 to 2 minutes of rest between sets.
- Train on three nonconsecutive days per week: Monday, Wednesday, Friday or Tuesday, Thursday, Saturday.

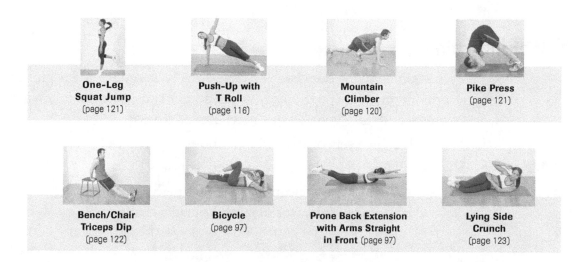

One-Leg Squat Jump (page 121) Push-Up with T Roll (page 116) Mountain Climber (page 120) Pike Press (page 121)

Bench/Chair Triceps Dip (page 122) Bicycle (page 97) Prone Back Extension with Arms Straight in Front (page 97) Lying Side Crunch (page 123)

Take It Up a Notch: For Advanced Exercisers

If you're able to perform the intermediate exercises with good form for the designated number of repetitions and sets, and/or you need a cardio boost, follow the instructions in this section for more challenging workouts.

Cardio

ADVANCED

- Warm up for 5 minutes
- Do 40 minutes of intervals: 4 minutes at 80 to 90 percent HR max, followed by 2 minutes of active recovery at 60 to 75 percent HR max.
- Cool down for 5 minutes.

- Do cardio five to seven times per week, following weight training or on alternating days.
- Total workout time, including warm-up and cooldown: 50 minutes.

Weight Training

In addition to the exercises you have already learned in the beginner and intermediate programs, you can add or substitute the following exercises to take yourself to a new level of fitness.

- Do three sets of 10 to 12 repetitions per exercise.
- Allow 1 to 2 minutes of rest between sets.
- Train on three nonconsecutive days per week: Monday, Wednesday, Friday or Tuesday, Thursday, Saturday.

Split Jump (page 128)

Elevated Leg Plank, Alternating Legs (page 128)

Lateral Box Jump-Over (page 129)

Flutter Kick (page 130)

One-Leg Squat Jump (page 121)

Back Extension on Stability Ball (page 114)

One-Leg Stability Ball Leg Curl (page 130)

Atomic Sit-Up (page 131)

Incline Reverse Crunch (page 107)

Pull-Up Using Body Weight Only (page 101)

Decline Twisting Crunch with Medicine Ball (page 107)

Diamond Push-Up (page 132)

Jackknife on Stability Ball (page 132)

Plank (page 122)

Stability Ball Push-Up, on Toes (page 133)

Lateral Foam Roll Jump-Over (page 134)

Take It Up One More Notch with Peripheral Heart Action (PHA) Training

Peripheral Heart Action Training is a variation of circuit training designed to work your cardiovascular system by alternating lower-body exercises with upper-body exercises. This forces the heart to work harder by having to shunt blood up and down the body to the working muscles. It differs from traditional circuit training because you will use moderate to heavy weights instead of lighter weights during a circuit. It can also be done with body weight only to create an amazing cardiovascular and strength workout. The benefits? You'll maximize fat burning and increase postexercise oxygen consumption. You will also get maximum cardiovascular and muscular endurance by keeping blood moving from one body part to the next, not allowing it to pool in any one place for a period of time. Here's how you do it: Take your current workout and order the exercises so that you have a leg or ab/lower-back exercise followed by an upper-body exercise. Repeat this technique with three sequences of four to six exercises. Do between 8 and 20 repetitions with no rest between exercises. You can rest for up to 3 minutes between sequences. The workout would look like this:

Sequence #1
- Dumbbell Squat: 10 to 20 reps
- Abdominal Crunch: 10 to 20 reps
- Push-Up: 10-20 reps

- Prone Back Extension with Arms Straight in Front: 10 to 20 reps
- Figure Four: 10 to 20 reps
- Dumbbell Pull-Over on Stability Ball: 10 to 20 reps

Perform the routine one to three times through depending on your fitness level, then move on to the next sequence.

Sequence #2
- Dumbbell Squat Jump: 10 to 20 reps
- Pike Press: 10 to 20 reps
- Leg Press: 10 to 20 reps
- Push-Up with T Roll: 10 to 20 reps
- Machine Abdominal Crunch: 10 to 20 reps

Perform the routine one to three times through depending on your fitness level, then move on to the next sequence.

Sequence #3
- Dumbbell Step-Up on Bench or Step: 10 to 20 reps
- Machine Triceps Push-Down with Rope: 10 to 20 reps
- Incline Reverse Crunch: 10 to 20 reps
- Dip: 10 to 20 reps
- Machine Lower-Back Extension: 10 to 20 reps

Stretch all muscle groups and hold each stretch for at least 30 seconds.

Adjust the Exercise Equation

Make it easier. If you feel the exercise is too hard on you, simply cut back the amount of time or the number of days you are doing or reduce the intensity. If you are doing 30 minutes of walking, cut back to 20 minutes, or any amount that makes you feel better. If your resistance training is too difficult, reduce either the amount of weight/resistance you are using, the number of reps you are doing, and/or the number of sets until you feel comfortable. Then continue to progress again at a comfortable pace. If you are a beginner, start with a beginner program, not with the more advanced ones. It will not help you to jump ahead. Be sure to write down the details of your daily workouts so you can track your progress. If you cut back or reduce your exercise, you must also cut out any reward foods.

Make it harder. If you are a beginner but find the beginner programs to be too easy, first try the progressions, then go ahead and move up to an intermediate program. As long as you can complete the workout safely, with good form and feeling good at the end, you're golden. If you're an intermediate, try some of the advanced workouts. Check out the box about PHA training on page 195.

Fine-Tuning the Food Formula: What to Do If You Want to Lose More

If you are eating all your meals and therefore all your daily calories, that's great. Do not, I repeat, do *not*, eat less. This will not help you lose more weight. Instead, either add exercise or increase the intensity of the exercise you are currently doing. To do this, choose one of the more difficult workouts if you are up to it. Or increase the intensity of your cardio by walking hills instead of flats; increasing the incline on the treadmill, stair-climber, or elliptical machine; or doing an interval program that I have mapped out for you in this chapter. But be sure to do only what you can handle. You can also think about trying a circuit training or a PHA type program as outlined in the sidebar on page 195.

If you're still hungry, run through this "debug" checklist and make sure you're doing everything right.

☐ I am eating all my meals and snacks.

☐ I am measuring my food to ensure the portions are correct.

☐ I am drinking at least 64 ounces of water a day.

☐ I am eating just the food on the list and not adding in other foods.

☐ I am getting at least seven hours of solid sleep per night.

☐ I am exercising for all the designated number of days.

If you did not check all of these, the next day do everything on the list and see if you are still hungry. If you are, consider adding either another snack or a recommended supplement, to help curb your appetite. Refer to chapter 5 for detailed information on what the supplements do and when to take them.

Body Emergency: One-Week Deadline

If you really have only a week and you need to lose some fat in a hurry, you can use this plan and then move on to another deadline. This is a five- to seven-day plan only! It is strict and the calories are very low, so staying on this plan for more than a week could wreak havoc on your metabolism and make you fatter. Bottom line: doing this any longer than a week is simply foolish. Also note that when you move on to another deadline plan, it may take a few days for your body to adjust from this one-week routine. So don't be upset if the scale goes up a tiny bit; it will come back down.

911 Eating Plan

You will eat five times per day regardless of your gender or weight. However, you will choose the appropriate portion sizes based on your gender and weight. Meals 1 through 4 will be the same for all weight ranges.

Women 128 pounds or less

- For meals 1 through 4, have a shake made with protein powder equaling 20 protein grams, 8 ounces water, 5 strawberries, blueberries, or raspberries, and 1 teaspoon flaxseed oil.

- Meal 5 will be the last meal of the day and must be eaten no later than 8 p.m. Choose 4 ounces cooked fish, chicken (white meat only), or turkey (white meat only); 1 cup any green vegetable; and 5 almonds, cashews, or walnuts *or* 5 black or green olives *or* 1 teaspoon of olive oil.

Women more than 129 pounds

- For meals 1 through 4, have a shake made with protein powder equaling 25 grams of protein, 8 ounces water, 10 strawberries, blueberries, or raspberries, and 1 teaspoon flaxseed oil.
- Meal 5 will be the last meal of the day and must be eaten no later than 8 p.m. Choose 5 ounces cooked fish, chicken (white meat only), or turkey (white meat only); 1½ cups any green vegetable; 5 almonds, cashews, or walnuts *or* 5 black or green olives *or* 1 teaspoon of olive oil .

Men 178 pounds or less

- For meals 1 through 4, have a shake made with protein powder equaling 38 grams of protein, 8 ounces water, 15 strawberries, blueberries, or raspberries, and 2 teaspoons flaxseed oil.
- Meal 5 will be the last meal of the day and must be eaten no later than 8 p.m. Choose 6 ounces cooked fish, chicken (white meat only), or turkey (white meat only); 1½ cups any green vegetable; and 10 almonds, cashews, or walnuts *or* 10 black or green olives *or* 2 teaspoons of olive oil

Men more than 179 pounds

- For meals 1 through 4, have a shake made with protein powder equaling 45 grams of protein with 8 ounces water, 15 strawberries, blueberries, or raspberries, and 2 teaspoons flaxseed oil.
- Meal 5 will be the last meal of the day and must be eaten no later than 8 p.m. Choose 8 ounces cooked fish, chicken (white meat only), or turkey (white meat only); 2 cups any green vegetable; and 10 almonds, cashews, or walnuts *or* 10 black or green olives *or* 2 teaspoons of olive oil.

911 Exercise Plan

During this week, your workouts will be limited to cardio only. This is the *only* plan that requires cardio exclusively, so don't confuse it with any of the other plans. Weight training is key to long-term success, but for this week your energy levels may be down, so cardio is the best way to burn a few extra calories without feeling exhausted.

Beginner

- Warm up for 5 minutes at 55 to 75 percent HR max.
- Do 30 minutes total: 15 minutes at 55 to 75 percent HR max, followed by 15 minutes of intervals of 3 minutes at 80 to 85 percent HR max, followed by 2 minutes of active recovery at 55 to 75 percent HR max. (See the box on page 195 for instructions on interval training.)
- Cool down for 5 minutes.
- Do cardio five to seven times per week, depending on your energy level.

Intermediate

- Warm up for 5 minutes.
- Do 40 minutes of intervals: 3 minutes at 80 to 90 percent HR max, followed by 2 minutes of active recovery at 60 to 75 percent HR max.
- Cool down for 5 minutes.
- Do cardio five to seven times per week, depending on your energy level.

Advanced

- Warm up for 5 minutes
- Do 40 minutes of intervals: 4 minutes at 80 to 90 percent HR max, followed by 2 minutes of active recovery at 60 to 75 percent HR max.
- Cool down for 5 minutes.
- Do cardio five to seven times per week, depending on your energy level.

What's Next?

Congratulations; you've conquered one of the most difficult deadlines in this book. Now it's time to move on to another eating and exercise deadline that is longer-term. If you still feel that you need to lose a few more pounds, simply choose another deadline chapter that meets your time goal. If you have lost all the weight you needed to on this two-week plan, move on to chapter 10 for maintenance. You will then learn what to eat, how much to eat, and when to eat, in order to keep your lost weight . . . well . . . lost. Since you have lost the weight you wanted to lose, you will have to calculate how many calories per day you will need to eat to maintain your new weight. So whether you choose another deadline at this point or you move on to maintenance, you will be instructed on how to figure out your necessary caloric intake. It's a whole new set of numbers (calories, protein, carbs, fat) for your meals.

Follow the exercise plans so that your basal metabolic rate will stay high and help you lose easier and more consistently. Remember, you will *look* a whole lot better than if you didn't exercise!

10

Your New Body— for Life

Dreams are what gets you started.
Discipline is what keeps you going.

—Jim Ryan

You've done the hard part. Now your goal should be to maintain what you've accomplished. You don't need a strict plan anymore, because you know the rules. You understand the kinds of foods you need to eat and when you need to eat them—no skipping breakfast and saving all your calories for a single big meal—and that you must exercise to maintain your "new" weight.

Although you're no longer on a short deadline, you're now on the final deadline—the rest of your life. And this deadline has some doable guidelines for maintaining the body you've created. It's not as tough, but you do need to keep yourself in check.

>>> Romina's Story

Over the years, I have gained a lot of weight. But I was in denial about how much. My wedding has put things into focus for me. I'm getting married next year, and I want to lose 50 pounds. That's my goal, to lose the weight slowly, over a number of months.

I never learned how to eat correctly, which is why I put on so much weight. Right after I met Gina, she told me something that has stuck with me. Gina explained that you can either eat to survive, or survive to eat. I realized that I had been surviving to eat. I love to eat. I always looked forward to my next meal, and food made me feel better when things weren't right.

Because I didn't know anything about eating right or how to change, I consumed way too many carbs. I'd eat a bagel in the morning, not knowing it was so high in carbs. I also ate out a lot, especially in the evenings, not paying any attention to portion size. I didn't exercise consistently at all. I might get motivated and go to the gym for a few weeks or get a workout video, then I'd get unmotivated and just stop.

Gina put me on an eating plan that was realistic and easy to follow. It has *this* much protein, *this* many vegetables, and *this* many carbs in correct portions. I was surprised that the food on the plan is pretty much all the foods I like. Because everything is so measured out, I have learned to prepare all of my meals, rather than eat out so much. Now that I cook for myself, I see that there are so many options beyond junk food and starch.

> 66 Gina explained that you can either eat to survive, or survive to eat. I realized that I had been surviving to eat. 77
> —ROMINA

For exercise, I walk for 30 minutes every day, and it has made a complete difference. I wear a pedometer, which has encouraged me to have a more active lifestyle rather than sit around. Walking has made me more energetic and given me new things to do with my time.

It's been almost three months, and I've lost 18 pounds. The tightness of my clothes has gone away, and I'm almost ready to try on wedding dresses. What's best about the diet is that I have the tools and the knowledge to take care of myself and stay healthy—and that's something that'll be with me forever. ❮❮❮

Know Your *New* Numbers

Readjust your numbers to figure out how many calories you need per day to maintain your new weight. This is your total caloric requirement—remember? I asked you to calculate this number in chapter 5. Here are the instructions again, so you don't have to turn back:

1. Use the online calculator in the tools and calculators section of my Web site, www.ginalombardi.com, to figure out your BMR—basal metabolic rate.

2. Figure out your total caloric requirement by factoring in exercise. BMR × activity level = TCR

Lightly Active	You engage in everyday normal activity only	1.3
Moderately Active	You exercise three to four times a week for at least 30 minutes each session	1.4
Very Active	You exercise more than four times a week for 30 or more minutes each session	1.6
Extremely Active	You exercise six to seven times a week for 60 minutes or more each session	1.8

So if your BMR is 1,490 and you're moderately active, multiply 1,490 by 1.4. You need 2,086 calories per day in order to maintain your new weight.

3. Since you are in the maintenance phase now, you don't need to calculate your adjusted total calories (ATC) to tell you what you can eat in order to lose weight.

I was going on a cruise with my husband and needed to lose 10 pounds pretty quickly, in a couple of weeks. I had been frustrated after the birth of my son that I couldn't get the rest of my baby weight off. By the time I met Gina I had given up. I had tried Body for Life, but I figured I'm forty years old, I've had a baby, and I don't have a lot of time in the day—this is a lost cause.

> **I figured I'm forty years old, I've had a baby, and I don't have a lot of time in the day—this is a lost cause. But to my surprise, with Gina, I lost weight phenomenally fast.**
>
> —BRIDGET

But to my surprise, with Gina, I lost weight phenomenally fast. We put together a diet that allowed me to plan my own meals from a list of foods she gave me. She increased the amount of protein and vegetables I ate, and cut out starchy carbs and sugar. Before that I wasn't very strict about my eating. I watched carbs and sweets, but not diligently. On Gina's plan I felt great. I was full and satisfied and never got that weak or headachy feeling or felt sick or tired.

What Gina offered was rapid results but without being on an unhealthy crash diet. Plus I feel like I've changed my eating for life. <<<

New-Body FAQ

What's the new eating game plan? What else can I have?

Turn to chapter 6, and follow the three-month plan. It's solid and doable with lots of food choices. I've worked with hundreds of people who have found this maintenance technique to be the easiest way to keep the weight off.

It works this way: you'll eat either four meals a day or three meals and two snacks. Basically, you can enjoy many of the things you love, as long as you eat them in appropriate amounts—

amounts that fit into your total caloric scheme for maintenance. Remember what got you into trouble in the first place to avoid going back to your old ways. It seems very simple . . . and it is! Again, you continue to eat all the healthy items on the lists but add in other things that you like as long as the carbs, protein, and fat fit into your total caloric requirement for the day. The more you familiarize yourself with the nutritional content of the foods you love, the easier it will be to know when and where to add them into your eating plan. For instance, if you want to add a banana, substitute it for another carbohydrate like a piece of bread. Or split them in two to equal the right amount of carbs for that meal (half a banana and a slice of toast, for example). If you choose to eat something that you know is way off base, you will have to remove one or two things of equal value somewhere else in the day. And as long as you exercise consistently, you will continue to improve the look of your body.

This doesn't give you carte blanche to eat whatever, whenever. Remember, you got out of shape in the first place by making bad choices. Now that you've gone through at least one deadline program, you learned enough to recognize your past mistakes. If you want a slice of chocolate cake, make it a sliver and don't eat any bread at dinner. This isn't hard-core physics, just common sense. You'll see that you don't have to suffer and give up the foods that you love if you control the portions and make up the damage somewhere else in the day or week.

What can I do to stay motivated over the long haul?

To maintain your focus, continually set short- and long-term goals for yourself and keep track of your progress. For example, if you have a new goal of running a 5K for charity, start by logging your miles per week as well as how fast you're running. Try to set a personal best every so often. If your new goal is simply maintaining the weight you've lost, give yourself 2 to 4 pounds of "living life" room to fluctuate (say around the holidays) before cracking down on the eating and exercise plans again. This way you won't allow yourself to slip back. The trick here is to *not* let yourself get so far off track that you have to start all over again. Have fun, but keep yourself on a short leash.

What should I do if I fall off the wagon?

If you're hanging off the side of the wagon, remember why you picked up this book and got on the program in the first place. The reasons you plastered on your refrigerator, your bathroom mirror, your rearview mirror in your car. Do you really want to go back there? If you derailed with the eating plan, the workouts or both, figure out *why* and fix it.

Choose the three-month eating plan (perhaps again) if you find that one most comfortable. Select another form of exercise that's more interesting to you. Mix it up with things like indoor rock climbing, ballroom dancing, martial arts, or another fun physical activity that'll allow you to learn a skill and also burn a lot of calories. You don't always have to be in the gym.

Why have I hit a plateau and how can I start losing again?

First of all, *don't panic*. Plateaus happen and they are easily remedied. The human body may have a few mysteries left, but I assure that you a weight-loss plateau is not one of them. These things may be the culprit if you hit a plateau:

- You have been on one of the short-deadline plans—one month, two weeks, one week—for more time than was recommended. Immediately go on the three-month plan to get your metabolism back into shape. Be patient as your body adjusts. A couple of pounds up will turn into several down in no time.

- You are increasing muscle tissue and losing body fat. In this case, congratulations! You are automatically creating a more efficient fat-burning machine. This is a good problem to have. So remember, although you may see no change or little change on the scale, your body fat is dropping and so are your inches.

- You are eating too many carbs or you are eating far, far off the general list. By now, you know what to do here. But in addition to getting yourself back on the program, be aware that packaged foods and restaurant foods often have many hidden carbs. Foods like milk, cheese, and even condiments like ketchup have a few grams of carbs. These things may not be a problem for most people, but if you are carb sensitive you will have to keep a close watch on them.

- You're not drinking enough water. If you don't drink enough, you'll retain everything you do drink. In fact, lack of water in the body is one of the most common causes of fat-loss plateaus. So drink up!

Can I ever go to fast food drive-throughs again?

I'm sad that I even have to answer this question at this point, but . . . "no" would be the politically correct answer. However, over the last couple of years the big fast-food chains have shown some improvement when it comes to healthier choices. If you're driving to Vegas and there's nothing for miles except a fast food restaurant, consider these choices to keep you on track:

- Chicken caesar salad (or any salad, for that matter,) with the dressing on the side. With chicken added to those that don't come with it.

- Grilled chicken breast protein-style (wrapped in lettuce and tomato)

- Flame-broiled burger protein-style (wrapped in lettuce and tomato)

- A kid's burger with just lettuce and tomato and half the bun

- Side salads, apple slices, egg patties

- Bottled water

Fight Holiday Weight Gain

No matter how dedicated you are to keeping the weight off, it's hard around the holidays. Stay strong and follow these survival strategies:

- **Make a plan.** In anticipation of a big family dinner, eat light in the morning with a lower-sugar fruit (like an apple or strawberries) and a couple of hard-boiled eggs. (But don't skip meals or you'll be ravenous later!) Don't fill up on hors d'oeuvres or other "pre-meal" temptations. When you pull up to the table, choose wisely: turkey (or other proteins) and vegetables over starchy choices like mashed potatoes and breads.

- **Work out in the morning.** Most gyms have limited hours on holidays. If yours is closed, plan to do a brisk walk or an in-home workout.

- **Don't party hardy.** When clients, friends, or family invite you over for drinks, less is more. Have one drink, then move on to a sparkling water. Four ounces of red wine or even light beer is a good choice if you keep it to a two-drink maximum.

- **BYOF.** If the festivities are not at your own home, offer to bring your own dish so that you can count on at least *one* choice that will be healthy and calorie controlled. Or find a calorie-free zone and sit, stand, and socialize as far from the food table as possible. Help do the dishes or move into another room for some good conversation without the temptations of desserts and lingering piles of decadent dishes.

- **Stay on track.** Continue to work with your trainer. In fact, schedule extra sessions for the weeks leading up to the holidays. Watch your favorite workout show and exercise along with it or rent a fitness video or DVD to stay mentally strong and connected to healthy choices.

An event's coming up—what advice can you offer about getting back on a "deadline"?

If some time has gone by and you feel you don't look quite as good as you did when you completed one of the deadline programs, jump back on to the one that suits your needs best. It should be comforting to know that you have this book to get you back on track if you've been slowly slipping. I understand that life gets in the way sometimes, but it's up to you to take care of yourself. If you have an event approaching, choose the appropriate deadline chapter to get you there and quickly get back on maintenance. It's that simple.

Eat and Run

Traveling, either for business or for pleasure, can send the healthiest intentions into a downward spiral. But even when you're on the road, it's important to stick to your guns. Here are some tips to keep you focused.

A little planning goes a long way. It's best to eat small meals and snacks throughout the day. So think ahead. Don't wait until you're starving: if you know you're going to be stuck on a flight with no meal service, pack something you can eat to prevent your blood sugar from plummeting and keep your cravings at bay. Best choices: celery sticks and a small container of peanut butter for dipping, string cheese and an apple, or a protein bar that has good whey protein and lower carbs (25 grams or fewer).

Plan even more. Bake a week's worth of sweet potatoes on a Sunday, cut them in half, and bring them to snack on along with hard-boiled egg whites or fat-free cheese sticks. They're portable, taste great cold, and are loaded with vitamins.

Choose lettuce. Wrap leftover chicken in a giant lettuce leaf and eat it anywhere a sandwich would work. Throw on some tomatoes and a drizzle of olive oil, and you've got a decent minimeal.

Be creative. Good food for road warriors includes cottage cheese, string cheese, celery, peppers, carrots, and apples. Throw some berries into a plastic container with some cottage cheese and nuts, and take it with you. In a pinch, high-protein, low-carb snack bars are better than vending-machine options.

Choose wisely in the air. Since most airlines do not automatically provide meals (unless you are flying first class), they often have meals for sale. Options usually include a fruit and cheese plate or some sort of salad. These would be your best choices. Forgo drinking alcohol and caffeine and avoid high-sodium snacks and drinks (pretzels, peanuts, Bloody Mary mix, V-8 juice) to minimize dehydration. Even better, bring your own food on board and order water, water, water.

Stay focused behind the wheel. Get plenty of rest before you hit the road and take frequent breaks so you can remain alert on the road and resist the urge for a caffeine fix. Stock up on good-for-you goodies so that you can motor past those fast-food joints that tempt you on the trip.

Go nuts. Nuts provide good fats, fiber, minerals, and a little protein. They also fill you up. The key is to not buy the big bags and nibble all day. Make your own little sandwich bags with a dozen or so nuts in each, and combine them with an apple or some string cheese. Best choices: walnuts, cashews, and almonds.

Hail (chicken) Caesar. At long last chicken Caesar salad has become a staple at take-out restaurants in airports. If you control the amount of dressing, it's a perfect meal. Buy it!

Order wisely. When eating out, choose fish, lean meat, or chicken, and a ton of vegetables. Skip potatoes or rice and double the veggies. Send the bread back, and for dessert, order fresh berries. Even if they're not on the menu, most places have them.

Refresh Your Workouts

By now, you're probably not a beginner anymore when it comes to training. And your body knows it. It's going to demand that you change things up frequently and work harder in order to stay fit and lean. If you've completed the beginner workouts, move on to the intermediate ones and then try adding some advanced exercises when you feel you are ready. But if you're already a more experienced exerciser, there are lots of ways to make your workouts more challenging:

Change the scheme of your exercises. In the deadline chapters I talked about making it harder and taking it up a notch (or even two notches), by adding cardio intervals or doing Peripheral Heart Action training. These are great ways to get creative with otherwise boring workouts and at the same time, improve your fitness level, your look, and your body composition.

Add new tools to your workout. By using stability balls, medicine balls, kettlebells, cones, ladders, Plyometric boxes (angled or straight), or wide or narrow handle grips for machine exercises, you can create an environment that is more difficult or simply more dynamic while doing some of the same exercises you were doing in your program during the weeks prior.

Go for a goal. Find a new challenge by training for an event like a walkathon, a minitriathlon, a skater marathon, or a bike or running race. Even better, find training partners to help you stay motivated and kick up the pace. Join a team or take a class.

Change your body position. This puts a whole new twist on an exercise. For example, if you're used to doing dumbbell bench presses on a flat bench, try them on a decline or incline bench. If you've been doing push-ups in the traditional military style, try placing your feet up on a bench to elevate the lower half of your body. This puts more resistance on your upper body during the movement. By making simple changes like these, you'll have hundreds of "new" exercises to play with.

On the Run? Try This Time-Saver Workout _____

If you have little time, no equipment, and not much room, do my 24 Workout. It's awesome and takes only about 6 minutes.

The 24 Workout

1. Warm up with two sets of 24 jumping jacks and 24 squats.
2. Do the following exercises and then repeat with no rest.

> 24 lunges on each side
>
> 24 push-ups
>
> 24 mountain climbers
>
> 24 bicycle crunches
>
> 24 step-ups on a chair or 24 wide-stance squats
>
> 24 V crunches

Don't Let Stress Make You Fat

Remember how in chapter 2 I described how sleep deprivation can make you fat? Being unrested puts stress on the body and triggers the release of cortisol. The fat cells located in your abdomen and around your internal organs are sensitive to this hormone. That's why you may notice fat storage around your midsection when you have prolonged periods of stress. This bulge not only looks awful, but also puts you at risk for diabetes and heart disease. A double whammy!

Here are five quick tips for reducing stress and beating the cortisol demons:

Exercise! Period. Hands down, the benefits are tremendous on all fronts.

Practice deep, slow breathing. Learn to do this by taking a yoga class or reading a book on yoga breathing. Or try this method I learned from my yoga teacher:

1. Place one hand on your chest and the other on your abdomen.

2. Breathe in slowly through your nose for a count of four.

3. Expand your abdomen first, then fill up your chest.

4. Slowly exhale completely through your mouth for a count of four, releasing the air from your chest first, then from your abdomen.

5. Repeat up to ten times and you will feel incredibly calmer and more relaxed.

Change your environment. Go outside; take a walk. This will allow you to gain a new perspective and take the edge off.

Laugh it off. Read a funny book or watch a funny movie. Hang out with a friend or a loved one who makes you laugh. This is one of my favorite things to do. Laughing changes your chemistry . . . in a good way!

Put it on paper. Get the stressful thoughts out of your head, out of your body, and onto paper. There is something very cleansing about writing things down. Then *do* something about it and throw away the paper.

I truly hope that you will keep this book on your shelf and refer to it whenever you feel the need. My personal goal was to educate you enough so that you will always have the ammunition you need to have the body that makes you feel good. And what you'll find is that maintaining that body is easier than you thought if you just keep these good habits in place. After all, as Kobi Yamada said, "Be good to yourself. If you don't take care of your body, where will you live?"

Index